IMAGES
of America

HEYWOOD HOSPITAL

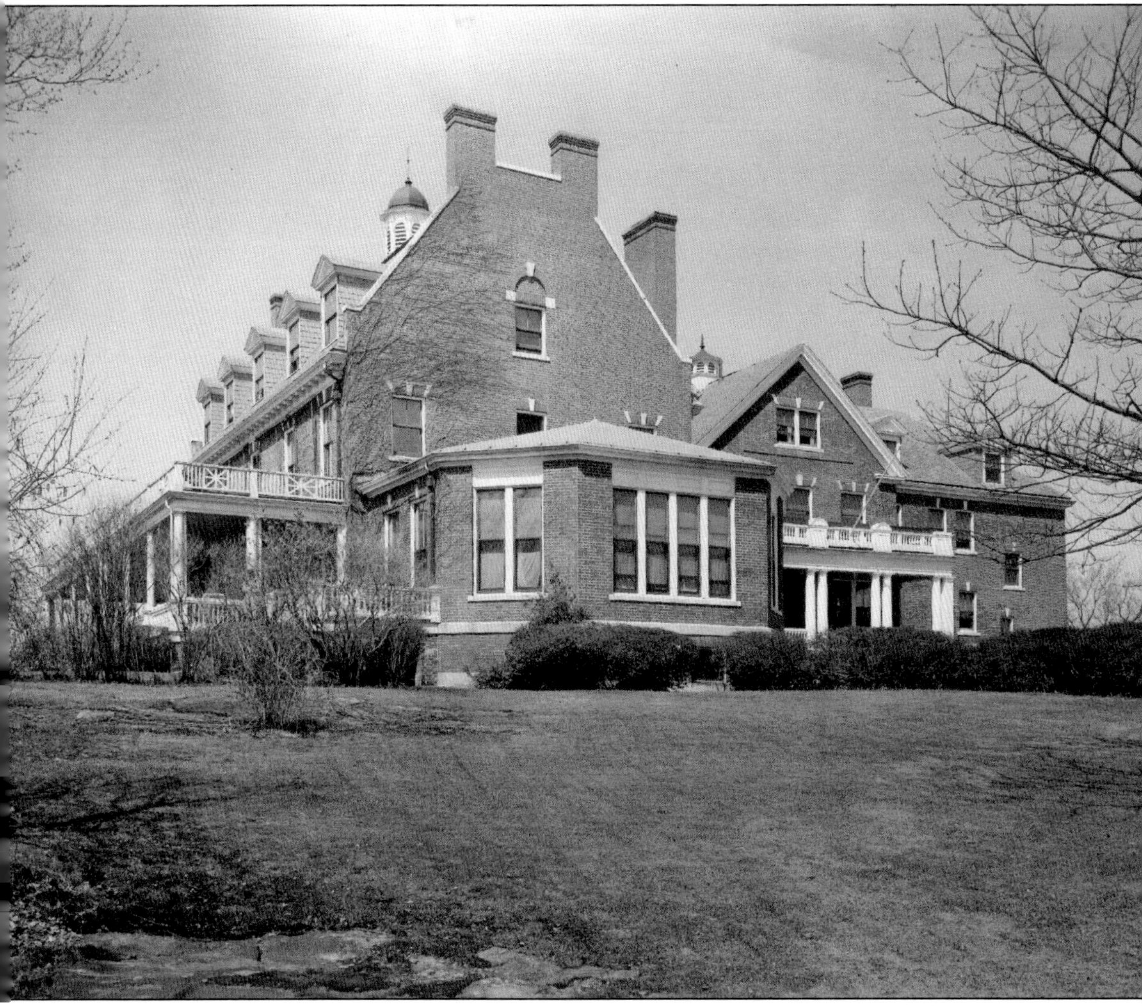

This image shows the Henry Heywood Memorial Hospital as it was originally built in 1907. Its architecture included breezy, white-pillared porches, cupolas, and stately chimneys. Situated on a hill overlooking Crystal Lake, the hospital afforded patients beautiful, expansive views of the lake to the west and of the then active Heywood family farm to the east. (Courtesy of the Levi Heywood Memorial Library.)

On the Cover: Taken in 1947, this photograph offers a nostalgic image of students of the Henry Heywood Memorial Hospital School of Nursing gathered in the Nurses' Residence around their music director and rehearsing for an event. Social gatherings were an important part of extracurricular activities. Sing-alongs were often incorporated into parties, teas, and other events, such as the much-anticipated capping ceremony. (Courtesy of Heywood Hospital.)

IMAGES
of America

HEYWOOD HOSPITAL

Gayle Kadlik and James A. Faust, MD

ARCADIA
PUBLISHING

ISBN 978-0-7385-7687-9

Published by Arcadia Publishing
Charleston, South Carolina

Printed in the United States of America

Library of Congress Control Number: 2011936769

For all general information, please contact Arcadia Publishing:
Telephone 843-853-2070
Fax 843-853-0044
E-mail sales@arcadiapublishing.com
For customer service and orders:
Toll-Free 1-888-313-2665

Visit us on the Internet at www.arcadiapublishing.com

To all who have been members of the "Heywood Hospital family" past and present—our patients, nurses, physicians, employees, volunteers, and donors—we thank you!

Contents

Acknowledgments

First, thank you to Heywood Hospital and its many departments for their support of this project. Without them, this book would still be only an idea. The Gardner Museum, Levi Heywood Memorial Library, South Gardner Historical Society, and Winchendon Historical Society were treasure troves of information and assistance. It is impossible to adequately thank all those individuals who contributed to the completion of this corporate history—at last count, almost 100! In typical "Heywood Hospital family" fashion, everyone jumped on the bandwagon to help out—from assisting technologically to digging up photographs, offering anecdotes, and so on. So, to all those who offered their encouragement, support, assistance, and/or contribution—you know who you are, as do we—please accept our gratitude!

Gayle Kadlik would like to give a special thanks to her husband, John, for his support throughout this undertaking.

Dr. James Faust would like to thank Heywood Hospital for allowing him to practice the full spectrum of traditional family practice for 38 years and dedicates his work on this book to Edward "Satch" Stromski, 1933–2011, a family man, athlete, exemplary volunteer, trustee emeritus, chairman of the board, and friend.

Images in this volume appear courtesy of the Gardner Museum (GM), the Levi Heywood Memorial Library (LHML), the South Gardner Historical Society (SGHS), and the Winchendon Historical Society, Inc. (WHS). Unless otherwise noted, the remaining images are from the archives of Heywood Hospital.

INTRODUCTION

Heywood Hospital is located 60 miles west of Boston in Gardner, Massachusetts, and only 15 miles from the New Hampshire border. The location and geography lend to a rich palette of vibrant autumn hues and challenging winter ski slopes. This land on which our forefathers fought and founded our nation is today often referred to as "Red Sox Nation."

Gardner has a rich history dating back to its early settlers, who came prior to the Revolutionary War. In fact, Gardner was named after Col. Thomas Gardner, who died fighting for his country at Bunker Hill. Once home to thriving chair manufacturers and considered the "Chair City of the World," Gardner has been transformed by economic changes and the outsourcing of manufacturing jobs into a commuter's city with Heywood Hospital as the major employer. As this book goes to press, Heywood Hospital employs over 1,000 people. Today, Gardner is a blue-collar community of 20,000 residents with proud ethnic backgrounds.

The history of Heywood Hospital portrays a grand metamorphosis over the last 100 years. In 1907, the hospital had 20 beds with four- and eight-bed wards. Today, the hospital has 153 beds with family-oriented, single-patient rooms. Likewise, as previously mentioned, the city of Gardner has undergone a metamorphosis from the Chair City of the World to a commuter city. In these times of consolidating hospitals, Heywood Hospital still serves Gardner as an independent, nonprofit community hospital.

Heywood Hospital was a gift to the city of Gardner from the Heywood family in memory of Henry Heywood. Heywood was the president of the Heywood-Wakefield Company during the time when it was the leading manufacturer of chairs in the world. Thus, the reader will be treated to the history of chair manufacturing in Gardner, including the original chair produced by James Comee, the first chair made by the five Heywood brothers, and the largest chair in the world.

The origin of Heywood Hospital began with Henry Heywood's wish that injured workers at his factory could receive medical treatment locally rather than having to travel to Boston. Upon his death in 1904, Heywood's wife, Martha, and daughter Helen fulfilled his wish by donating the land and hospital building in his memory. How proud he would be to know that today, over 100 years later, Heywood Hospital continues to serve area residents, allowing them to remain in their community for medical care.

An extra benefit to Heywood Hospital's centennial celebration in 2007 is that it brought together a rich collection of historic photographs and ephemera chronicling the fascinating history of the hospital. Through this walk down memory lane, members of the Heywood Hospital family—physicians, employees, patients, volunteers, and community members—are seen in their various roles throughout the years. Images such as the original architectural floor plans of the 1907 hospital are revealed. Photographs of early equipment, folks at work and play, and hospital celebrations provide a nostalgic glimpse into the past.

During the 1920s, the community's growing needs led to an expansion of space and services. Over the course of the 20th century, there were many major additions. The first of these additions was donated by Helen Heywood in 1926 and is known as the West Wing. The West Wing was primarily for child and maternity care. Next came the North Wing from 1941 to 1945 during the World War II years when many of Heywood Hospital's physicians rendered their service to the war effort. This wing housed a cafeteria and kitchen plus two medical and surgical floors.

This history of Heywood Hospital includes the Henry Heywood School of Nursing, established in 1926. There were 10 young women enrolled in the first nursing class, a three-year diploma program. A total of 638 students graduated in the school's 41 years of existence, which leads to wonderful stories. The disaster drills held at Heywood Hospital were at times partnered with the military and were nationally recognized. Likewise, the history of ambulances provides interesting images of early vehicles.

Another large project was the Favor Wing, named after a philanthropist with a soft heart for the poor. This four-floor expansion built in the 1960s and 1970s housed a new emergency room, surgical suite, medical surgical floors, telemetry, and intensive care unit. Advancing technology dictated an additional expansion—a new radiology wing. A photographic history of radiology reveals this advancement in machines and technology and the building of the new department. In 1970, a new kitchen and cafeteria fulfilled the dream of the first CEO. An increase in medical staff made it evident that a place to gather and interact socially and professionally was in order. The Pierce Conference Room was born and not only represented a memorial to an outstanding patriot and surgeon, but also acted as a catalyst for physician-community sports events.

Readers will enjoy images and an account of Winchendon Hospital and its eventual affiliation with Heywood Hospital. In 1990, the medical office building was funded, built by physicians, and opened for business.

The 21st century continued to bring growth to Heywood Hospital. The 2001 LaChance Maternity Center is humorously compared to the 1907 and 1926 obstetrical units. The new Ambulatory Acute Care Center of 2001 housed oncology, surgical day care, special procedures, and post-anesthesia care units. A look toward the future reveals the Center for Wound Care and Hyperbaric Medicine, the Watkins Center for Emergency and Acute Care, and a peek at the electronic intensive care unit.

While Heywood Hospital was undergoing multiple additions, the city of Gardner was going through its own transformation. Because of poor economic times and the outsourcing of manufacturing business, Gardner lost its furniture factories and became a commuter community. In spite of this, the community has remained engaged in supporting Heywood Hospital. This long-standing partnership for the common goal of maintaining an independent community hospital has remained steadfast and is filled with individual and organizational efforts that have all contributed to this mission.

We are pleased to present this collection of historical images and information about Heywood Hospital. We hope that this history of a small community and its hospital so richly connected to one another will be enjoyed by all.

One

Chair City

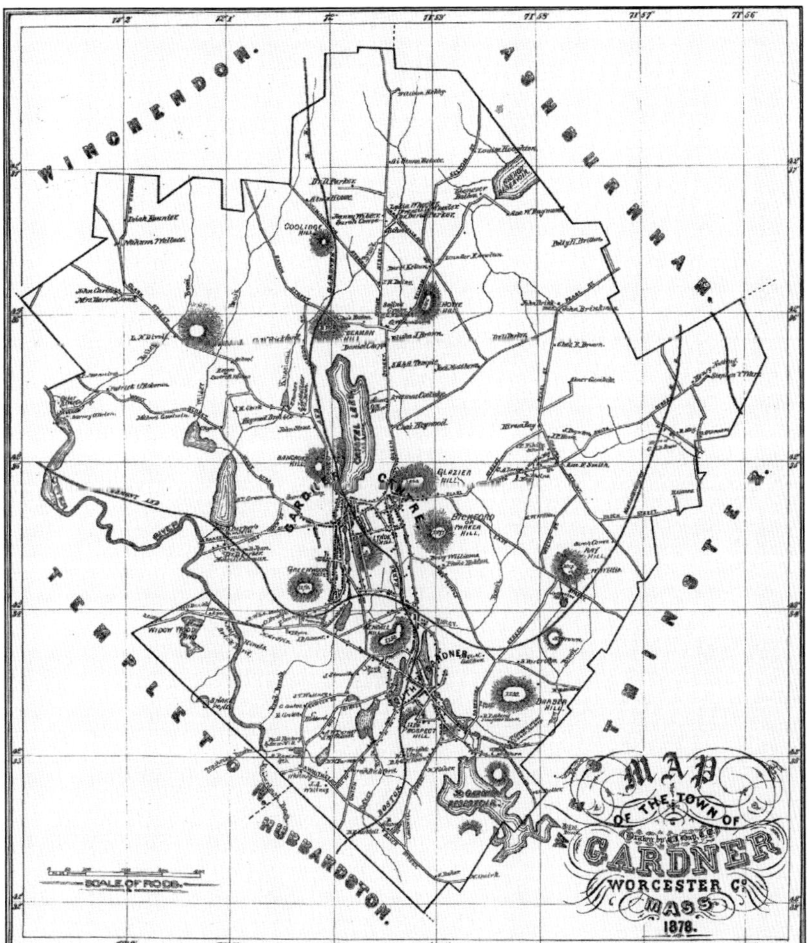

The history of Heywood Hospital cannot be properly told without first introducing a brief history of Gardner, Massachusetts. Both histories illustrate a strong sense of connection with community. Located in the north-central part of the state, Gardner received land grants from the towns of Ashburnham, Westminster, Winchendon, and Templeton and was incorporated as a town in June 1785. (Courtesy of SGHS.)

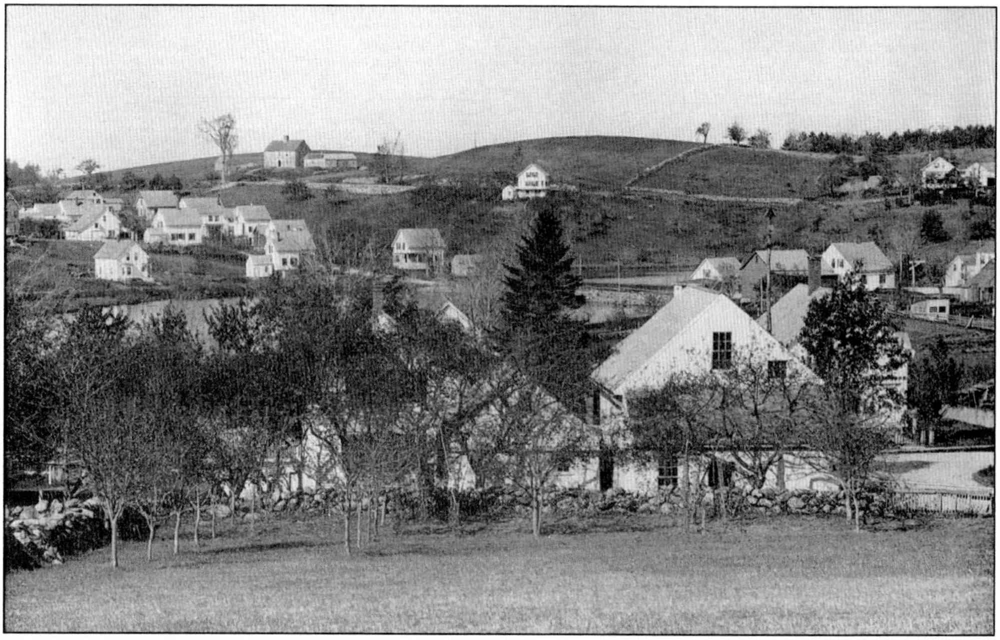

Elisha Jackson was the territory's first settler, preceding Gardner's incorporation as a town. He built his home, the Jackson Tavern, on the stagecoach road to Boston in 1764. A patriot, Jackson's name is on a list of citizens pledging not to buy tea from England. He went on to serve in the Revolutionary War as a captain. He also served his community by drawing up a petition to the Commonwealth of Massachusetts in 1785 to form a town so that the people could have their own meetinghouse and place of worship. When the petition was accepted, the town rewarded Jackson with the honor of town moderator. The image above shows the Jackson home in the mid-1800s on top of the hill at upper left. Below is an image of a float in the town's sesquicentennial parade in 1935. (Above, courtesy of LHML; below, courtesy of GM.)

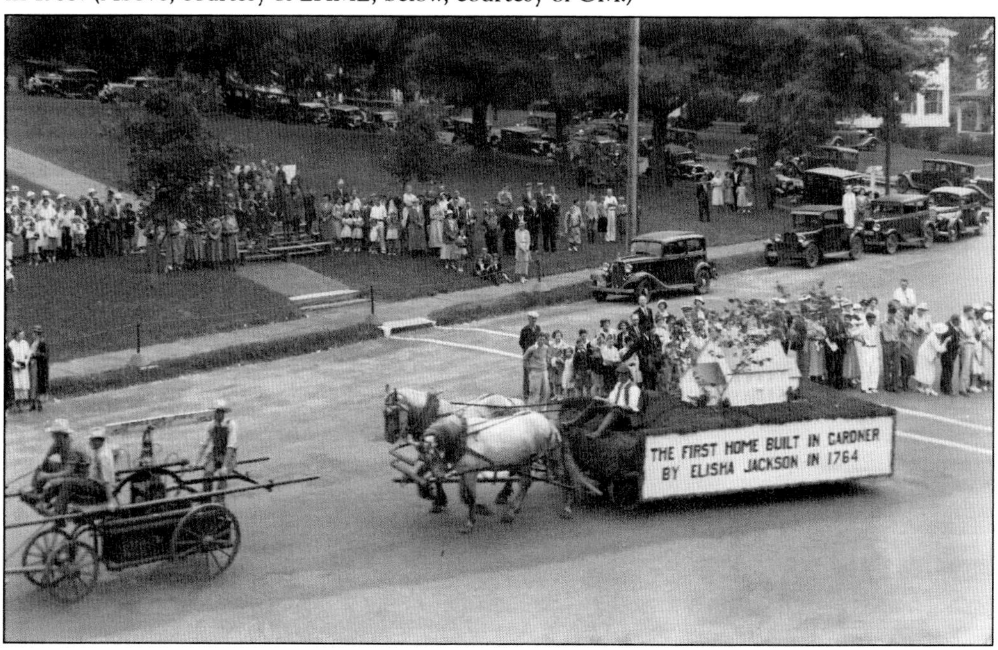
THE FIRST HOME BUILT IN GARDNER
BY ELISHA JACKSON IN 1764

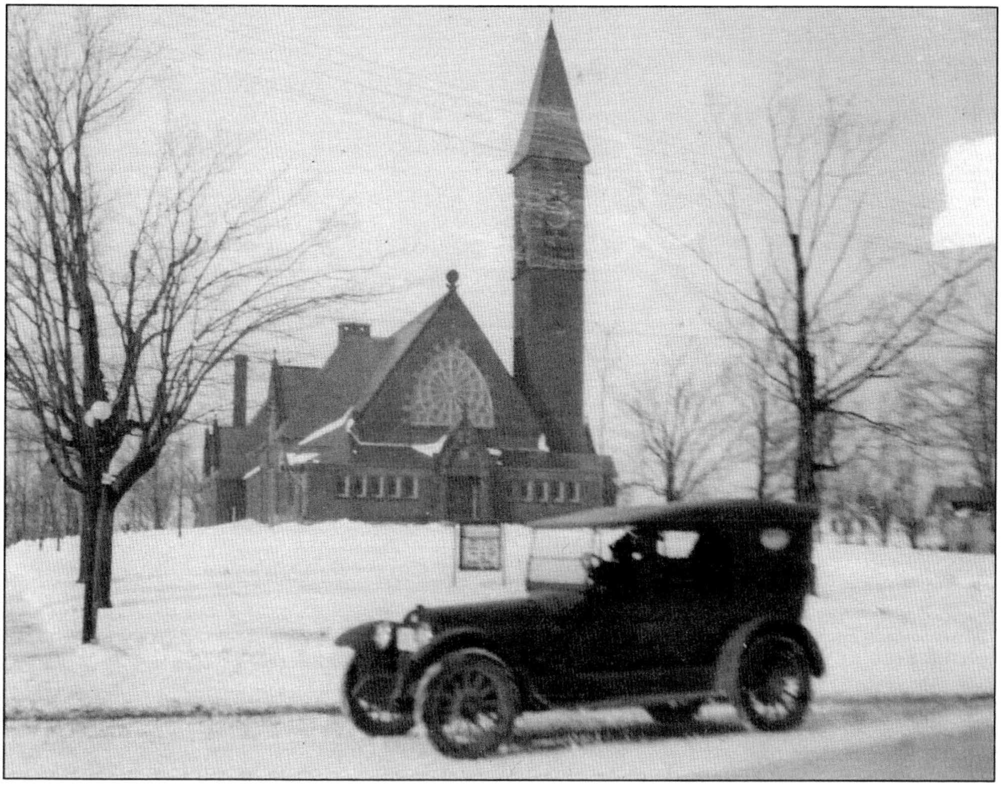

As was the law at the time, the residents of Gardner now had to undertake the task of building a meetinghouse. The town purchased four acres of land from Seth Heywood in 1786 for the purpose of a meetinghouse, a town common, and a burial ground. The First Congregational Church took four years to complete. In 1845, a bell tower was added, and the church became known as the Bell Meeting House. This building was eventually relocated and later burned. In 1878, a new church was built on the original site and is still standing with its own clock and bell tower, seen in the photograph above taken about 1930. Below is a view of Gardner in the late 1880s looking west, with the church and its steeple seen rising above the other structures. (Both, courtesy of GM.)

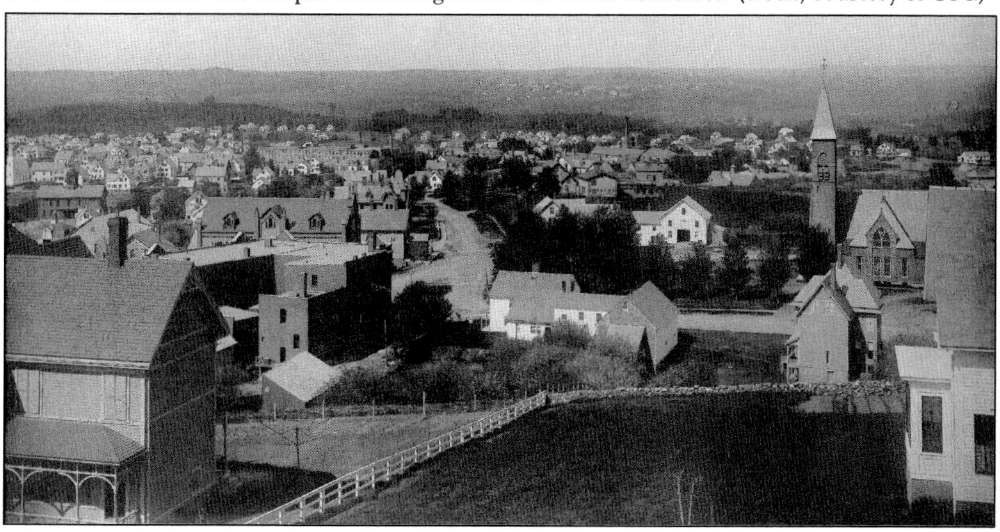

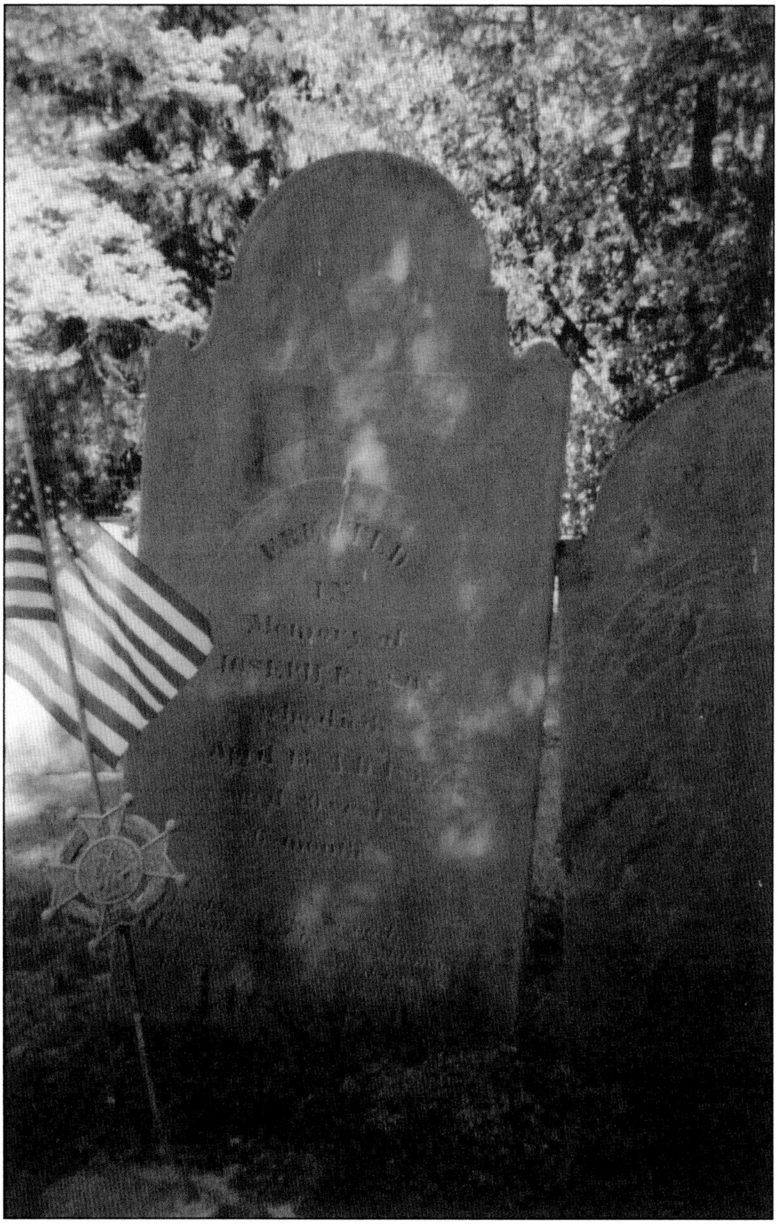

The spit of land that lies directly in front of the First Congregational Church is what remains of the old town common. Directly behind the church is the old burial ground. Proud of their newly found heritage, the residents of Gardner named their town after Revolutionary War hero Col. Thomas Gardner, who died from wounds received in the Battle at Bunker Hill. A social equal of John Hancock, Samuel Adams, and other early American heroes, Gardner's last words to his son from his deathbed were "Conquer or die!" Several early settlers of the area were also present at this infamous battle, including Seth Heywood. Many of the gravesites in the old burial ground adjacent to the church belong to veterans of the Revolutionary War and signers of the petition to form the town of Gardner. Seen here is the grave of Boston Tea Party participant Joseph Payson. Elisha Jackson, the territory's first settler, is also buried here. The first to be buried in this graveyard was one-year-old Sarah, daughter of the first minister and physician John Glazier.

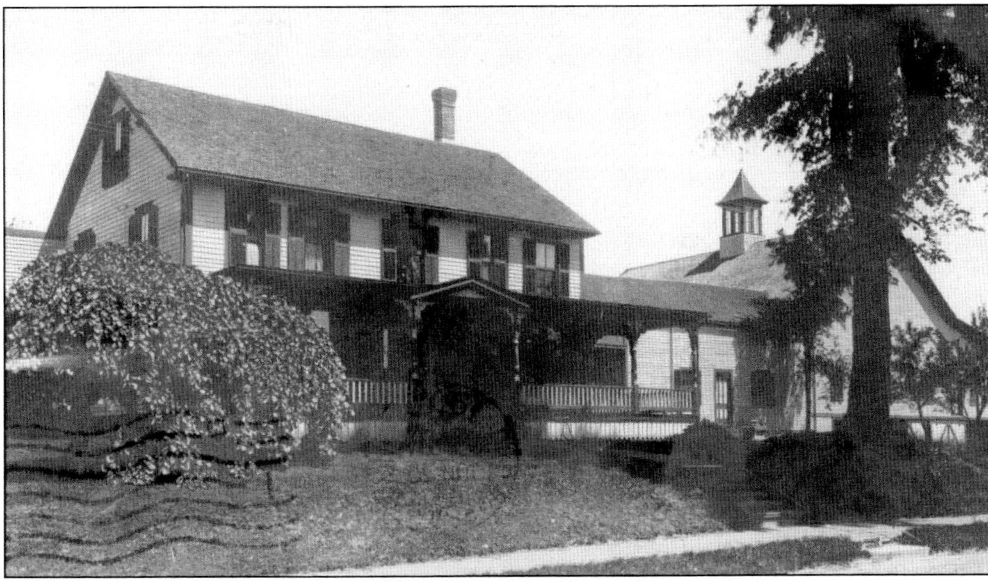

Located at 162 Pearl Street, the home shown above was built in 1774 by David Comee. His son James is attributed with founding the chair manufacturing industry in Gardner in about 1800 when he handcrafted his first wooden chair in this house. Horse-drawn wagons delivered his chairs to customers as far away as Boston. As his business grew, Comee hired and trained apprentices. Some of these young men went on to establish their own chair-making businesses in town. James Comee surely was instrumental in Gardner eventually becoming known as Chair City of the World. The chair shown at right was handcrafted by James Comee in 1800 and is displayed in the Gardner Museum today. (Above, courtesy of SGHS.)

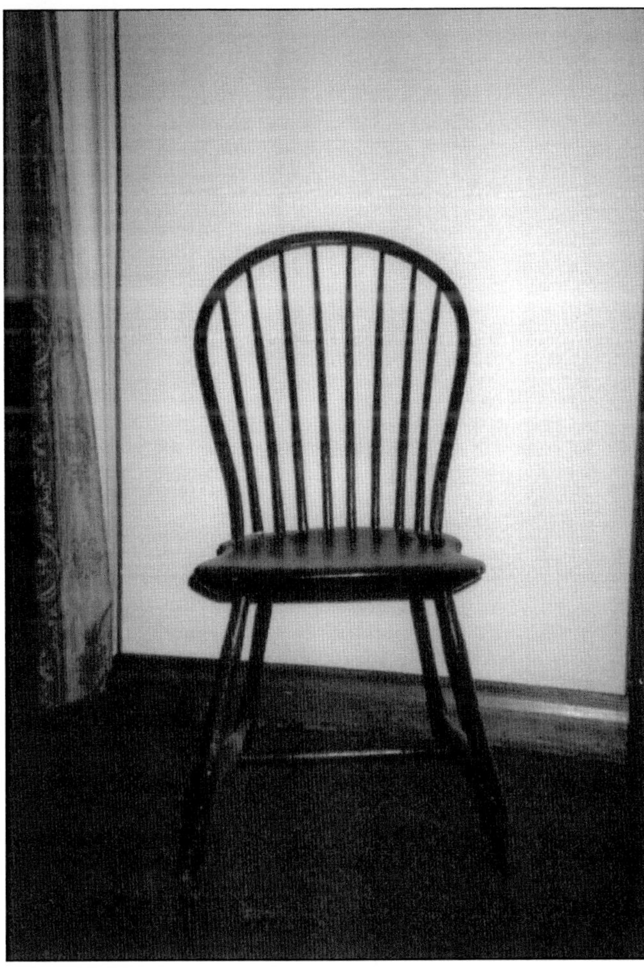

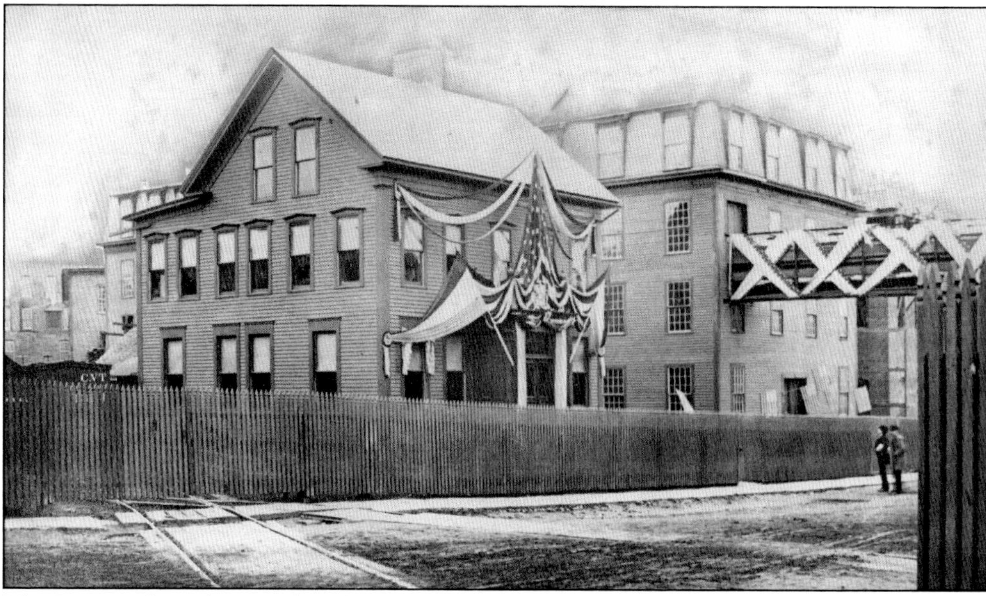

The Heywood Brothers and Wakefield Company, once the largest furniture manufacturer in the world, had its modest beginning in Gardner, Massachusetts. In 1826, the five Heywood brothers—Levi, Benjamin, Walter, William, and Seth—began making chairs in their father's shed on the corner of Elm and Central Streets. Thanks to the foresight of Levi, the oldest brother, the company was on the cutting edge of manufacturing and utilizing the very latest in machinery, such as circular saws, by mid-century. A series of catwalks, as seen to the right in the image above, connected various buildings to aid employees in moving between them. The last two catwalks were removed in 2006 for safety reasons. They were listed in the National Register of Historic Places. The image below shows a horse-drawn wagon used by the company to deliver chairs to customers. (Both, courtesy of LHML.)

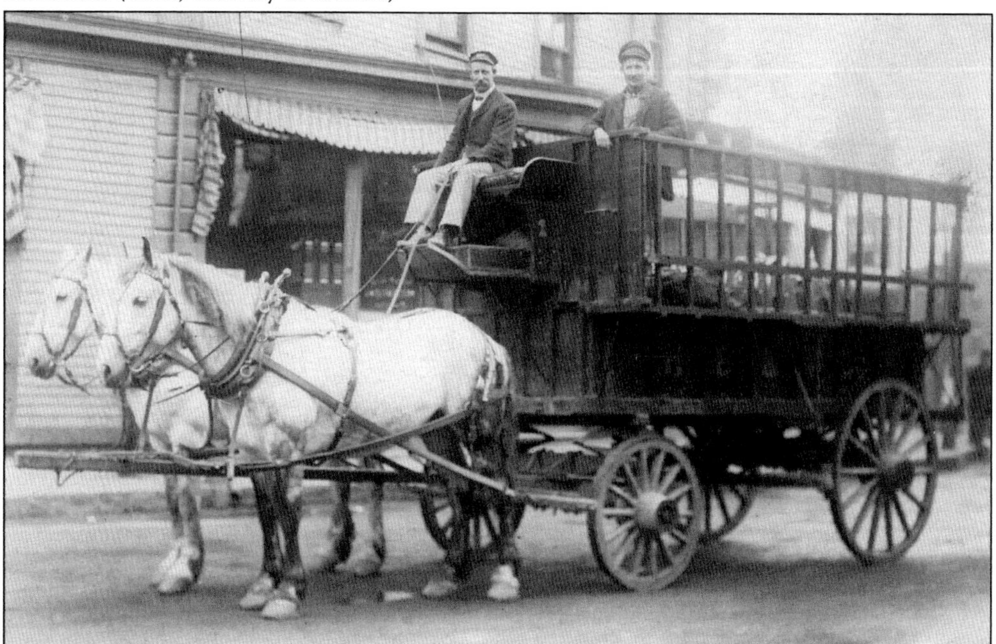

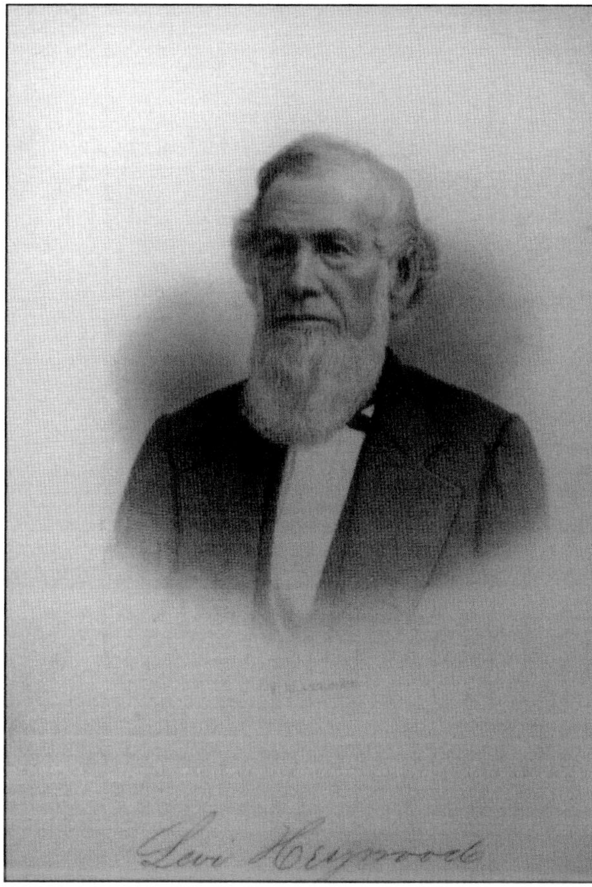

Levi Heywood is pictured at right in the mid-1800s. A pioneer in the furniture industry, he was considered a visionary by many. During his lifetime, Heywood and other townspeople had been interested in planning a town library. Following his death, his descendants bequeathed the Levi Heywood Memorial Library to the town of Gardner. Established in 1885, today it is the home of the Gardner Museum and is located on Pearl Street diagonally across from where Levi and his brothers constructed their first chair. Interestingly, a close look at the photograph below reveals the outline of a chair on the front facade. (Both, courtesy of GM.)

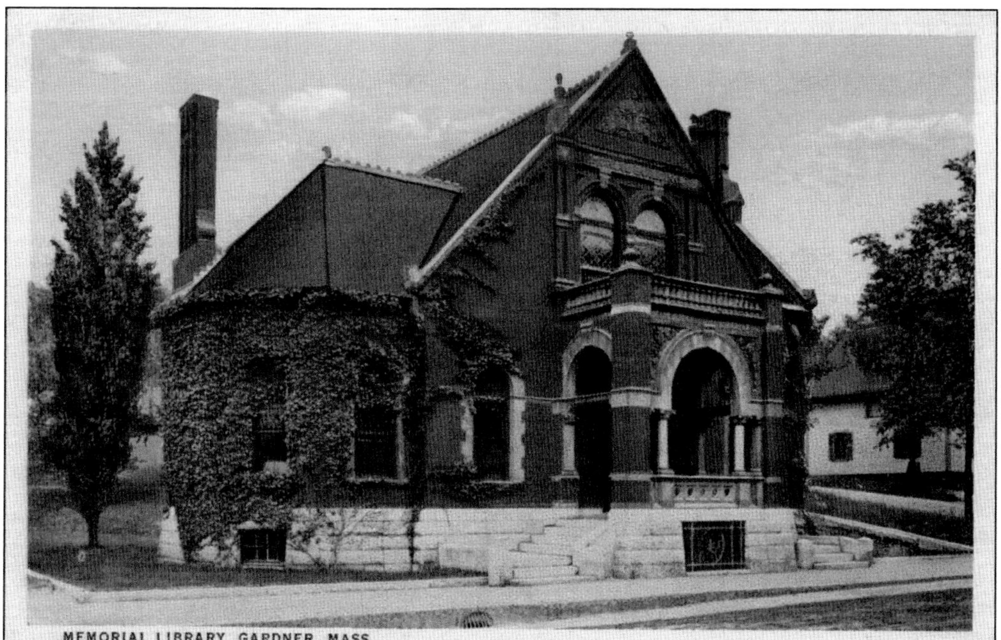

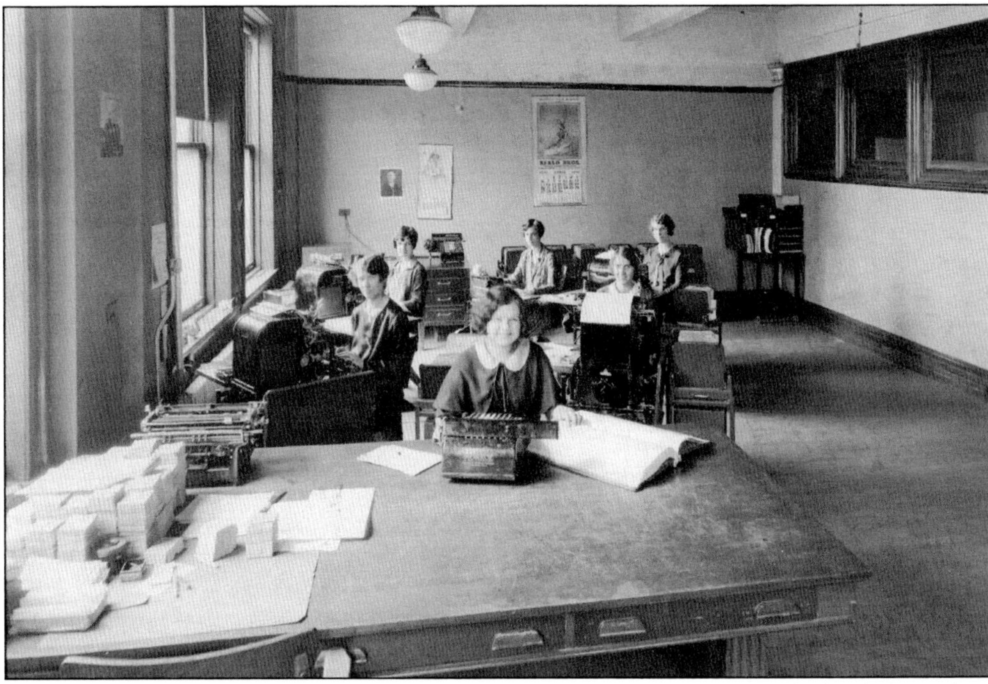

In the late 1800s, Edward G. Watkins invented one of the first punch time clocks while working as chief engineer for Heywood Brothers and Company. He went on to found the Simplex Time Recorder Company in Gardner, which became the town's prime employer after the decline of the chair industry in the 1950s. The Great Wall of China is secured by Simplex Time Recorder equipment. The company has since been sold. Today, Watkins's grandson Edward G. "Chris" Watkins II is a major supporter of Heywood Hospital. Above is a photograph of office workers employed at Heywood-Wakefield Company in April 1930. They are identified as Emilienne Leger, Jeannette Tousignant, Myrtle Fisher, Grace Gardella, Esther Bowin, and Olga Uppgard. Below is an image taken in 1935 during Gardner's eight-day sesquicentennial celebration. (Both, courtesy of GM.)

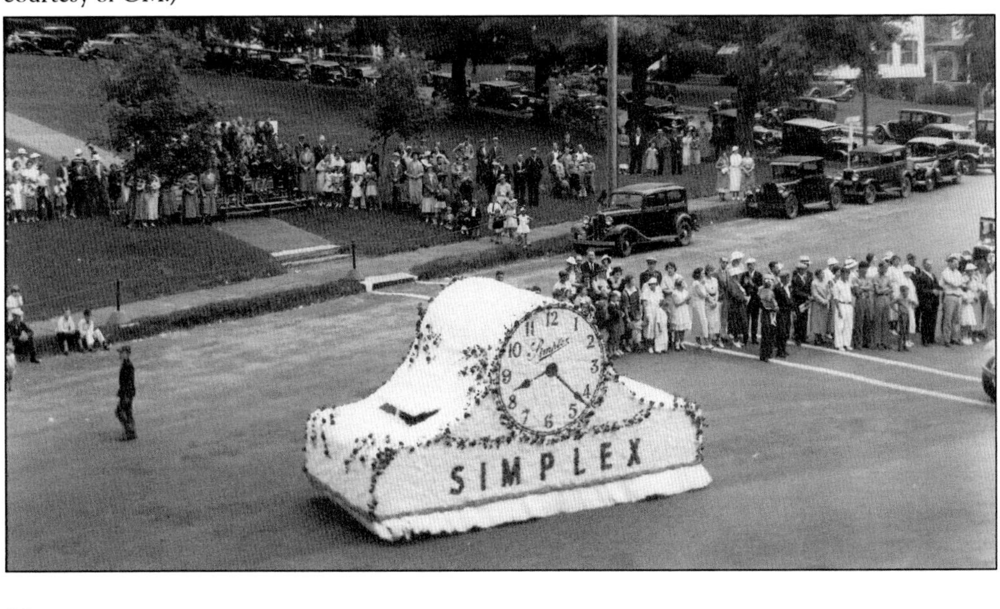

It was only fitting that Chair City of the World laid claim to the largest chair in the world, which was made by P. Derby and Company. Philander Derby arrived in Gardner around 1863 and began manufacturing chairs in a factory on Main Street. This mission-style chair weighed 1,200 pounds, stood 12 feet high, and used 600 feet of lumber. It stood for many years at Union Square. (Courtesy of GM.)

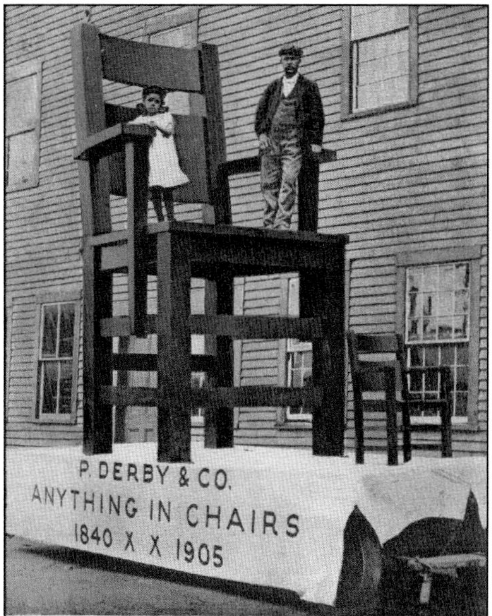

Biggest Chair and Man who made it, At Derby's Shop, Gardner, Mass.

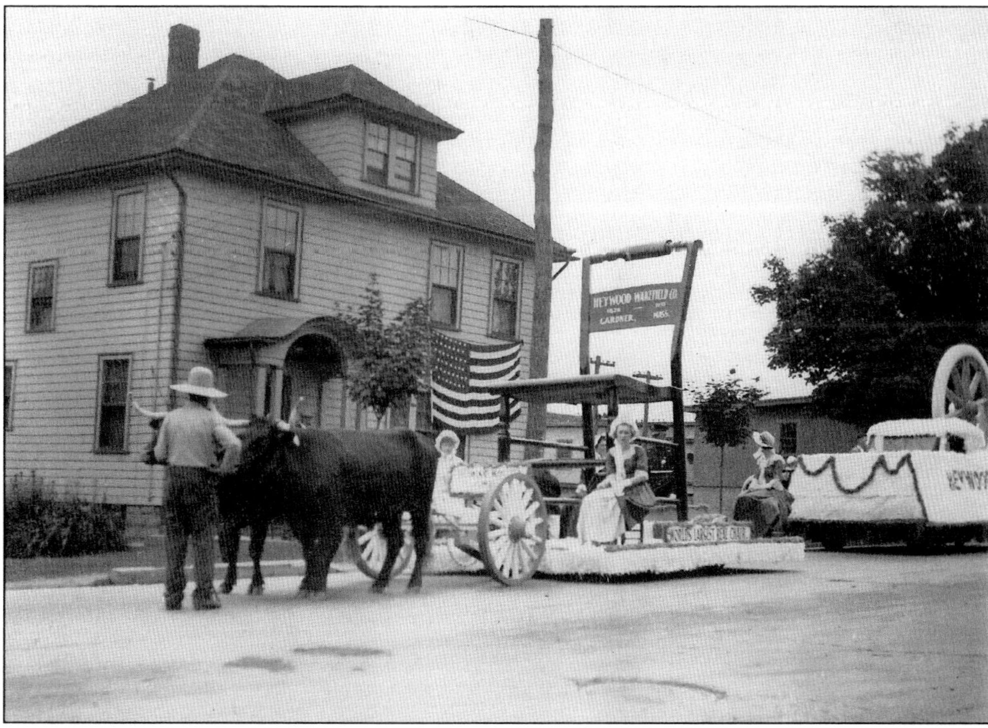

In 1935, the Heywood-Wakefield Company crafted the largest chair in the world. A reproduction of a Hitchcock colonial-style chair, it stood 13 feet, eight inches tall. The chair was first displayed in Gardner's sesquicentennial parade on a float drawn by a pair of oxen. It was then placed on the corner of West Broadway and the Mohawk Trail but was later moved to Gardner Center. (Courtesy of GM.)

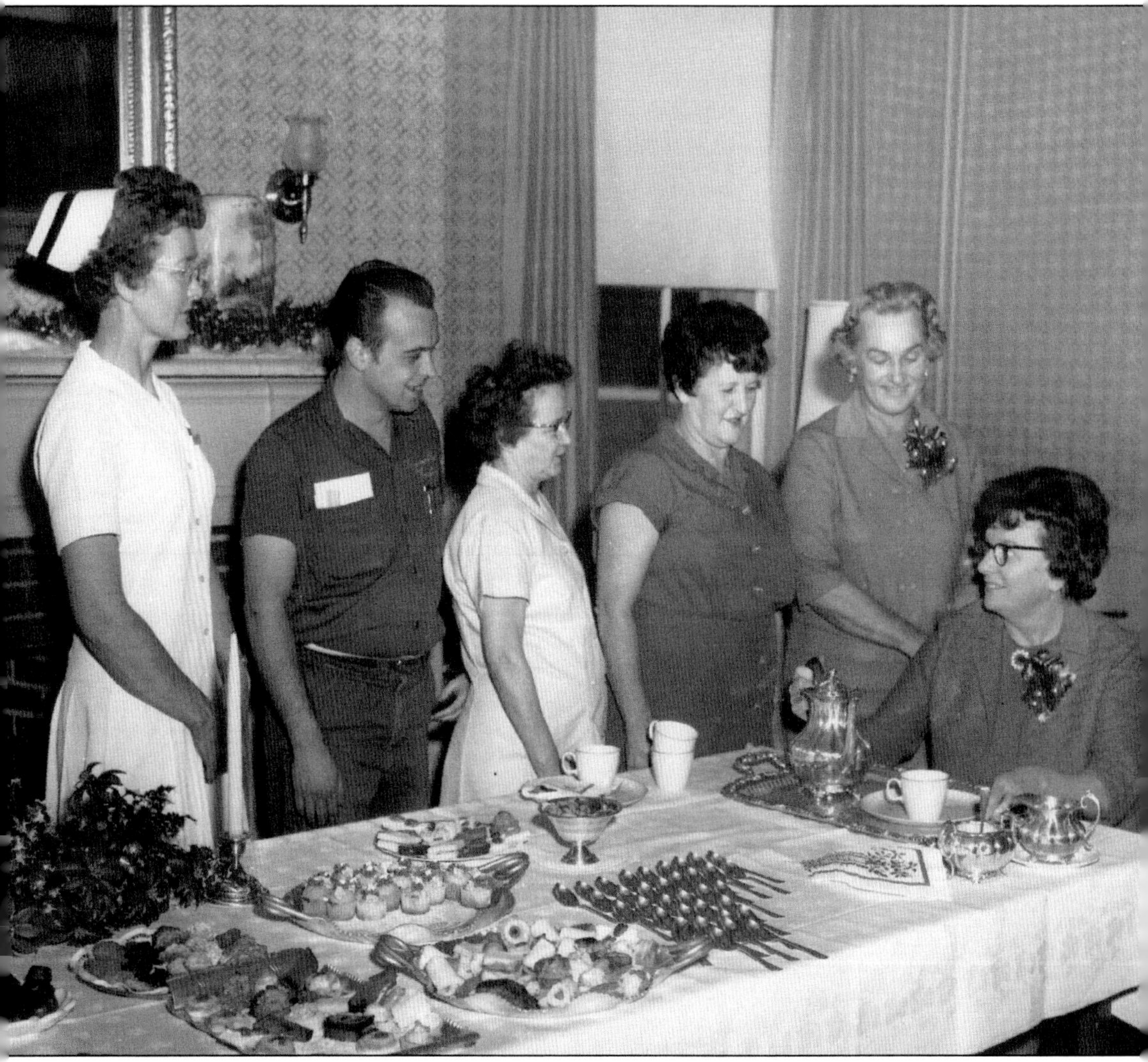

Although Gardner, Massachusetts, was certainly best known as the furniture capital of the world, it was also known for producing some of the finest hand-wrought and manufactured sterling silver goods in the country. The city's rich history as part of the silver industry began in the late 1800s when Frank Smith began to manufacture high-grade silverware. Arthur Stone, widely considered the dean of American silversmiths, opened his shop in Gardner in 1901. Throughout the 20th century, apprentices at these shops branched out to establish their own silver businesses. Today, popular silver pieces are still fashioned in Gardner by silversmith Peter Erickson, grandson of George Erickson who apprenticed under Stone. Pictured here is a silver tea service used only on special occasions. It is being used for a Christmas tea in the Nurses' Residence in 1967.

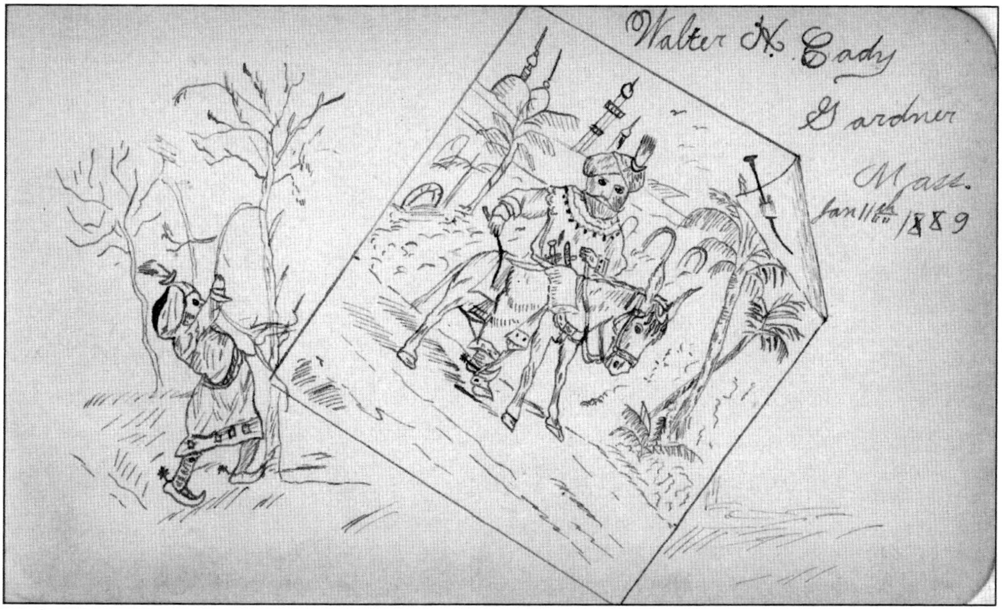

Walter Harrison Cady was born in Gardner, Massachusetts, in 1877. At 18 years of age, Cady left Gardner for New York City to embark on a lifelong career as an illustrator. He is perhaps best known as the illustrator of Thornton Burgess's bedtime stories for children or his own *Peter Rabbit* comic strip. Recently discovered and published here for probably the first time ever is a sketch by Cady in 1889 when he was about 11 years old. Donated to the Gardner Museum by a childhood classmate, the sketch in the autograph album was recognized by museum committee members cataloguing the item. At age 21, Cady designed the town seal for Gardner. Below is a plate depicting the seal, which credits the towns of Ashburnham, Westminster, Winchendon, and Templeton for their contribution of land. (Both, courtesy of GM.)

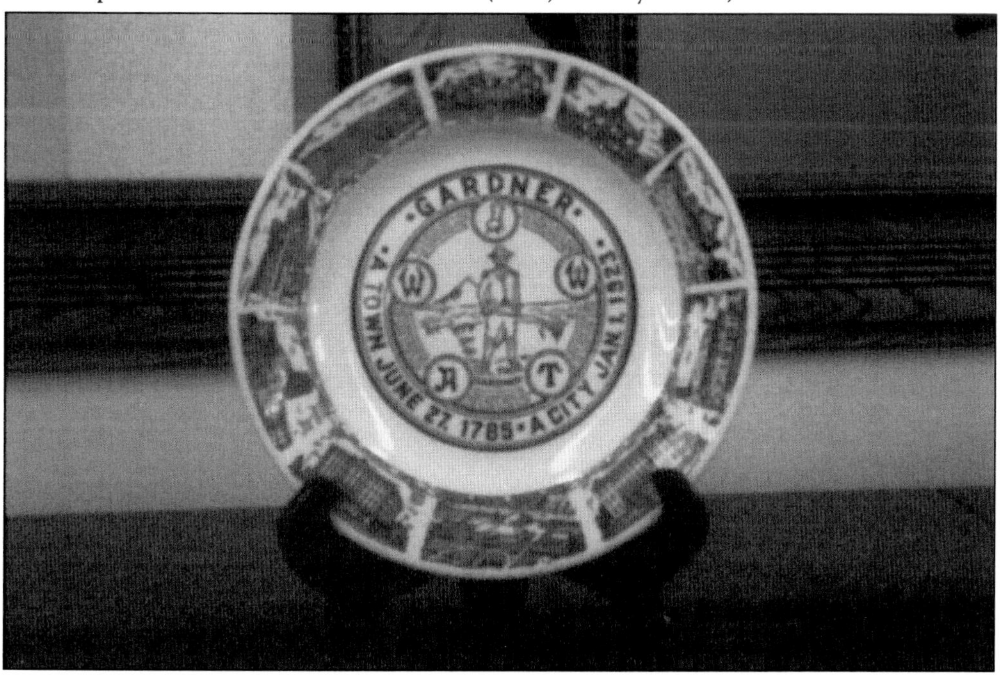

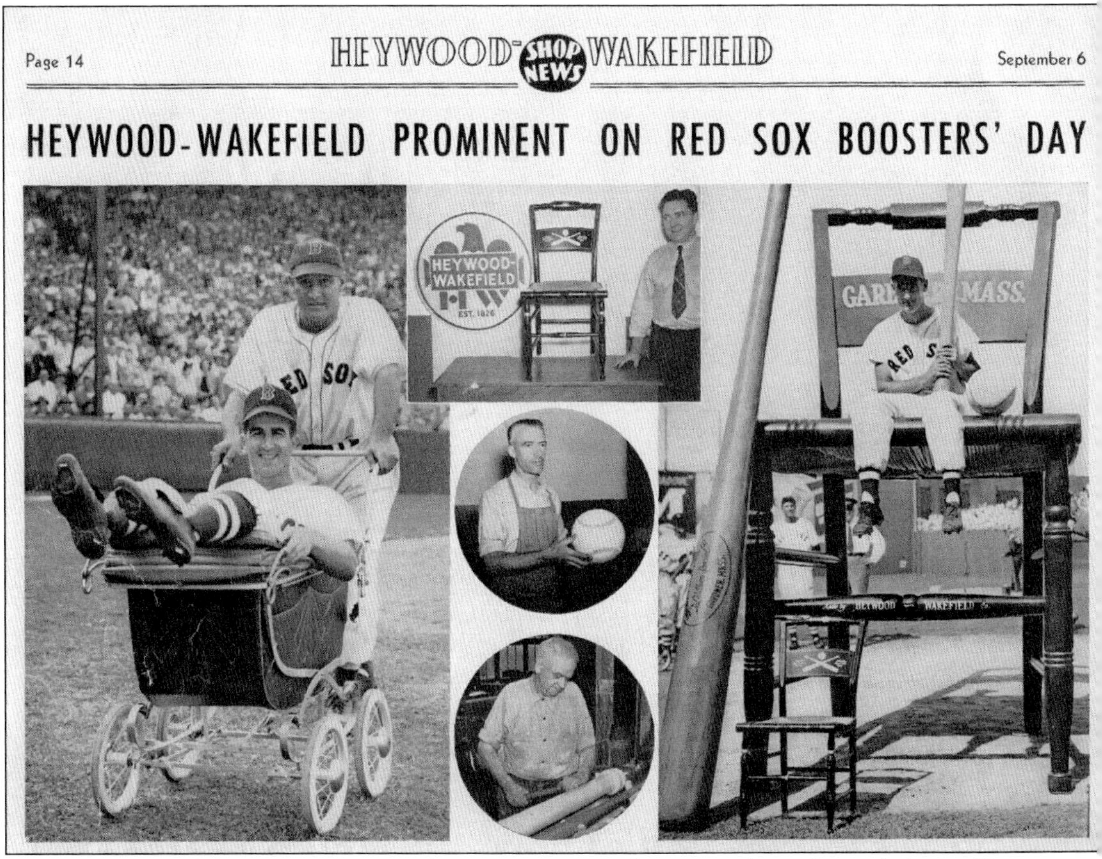
Page 14 HEYWOOD-SHOP NEWS-WAKEFIELD September 6

HEYWOOD-WAKEFIELD PROMINENT ON RED SOX BOOSTERS' DAY

Gardner made history once again when an entourage of 2,000 residents descended upon Fenway Park in Boston, Massachusetts, on August 25, 1946. With Gardner mayor Oscar R. Anderholm and Massachusetts governor Maurice Tobin doing the honors, the group presented Boston Red Sox home run hitter Ted Williams with the largest chair, largest bat, and largest baseball ever seen. In addition, each player was given a chair, a tricycle if a father, and a baby carriage if an expectant father. None other than Ted Williams had his photograph taken seated atop the chair and holding the bat and ball. The entire Red Sox team lined up for a photograph illustrating the huge dimensions of the bat. Photographs were seen in newspapers across the country, including in *Life Magazine*. Today, the bat holds a proud place at Cooperstown's Baseball Hall of Fame. With the cheering from an extra 2,000 fans, the Red Sox won both games of the double header that day. (Courtesy of GM.)

Two

The Heywood Family's Gift to the Community

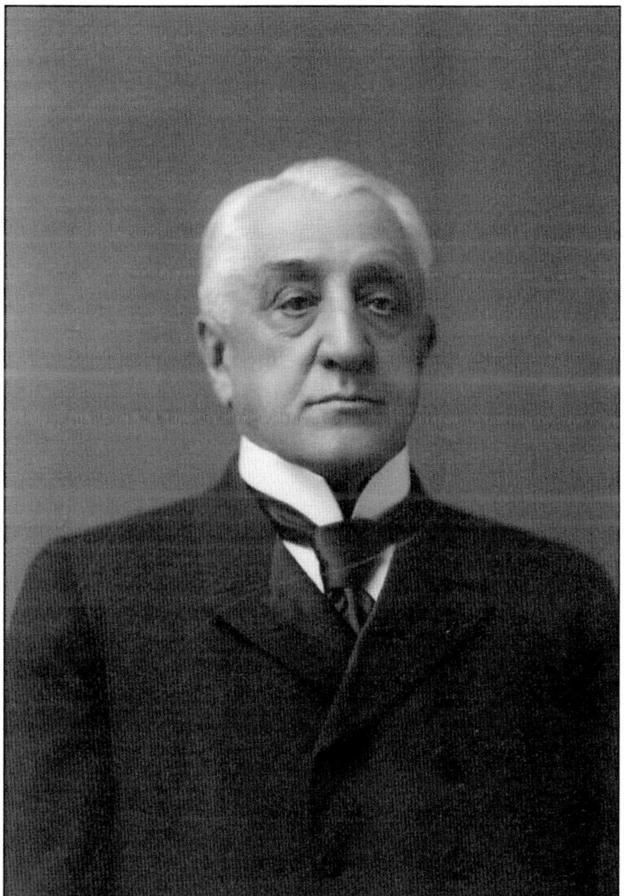

Henry Heywood was born in 1836, grandson of Seth Heywood, one of Gardner's earliest settlers. He married Martha Temple and had two children, George—who died at age 36—and Helen. In addition to his role in the family furniture business, Heywood was also a gentleman farmer and ran the Heywood Farm. He died in 1904 at age 68. (Courtesy of LHML.)

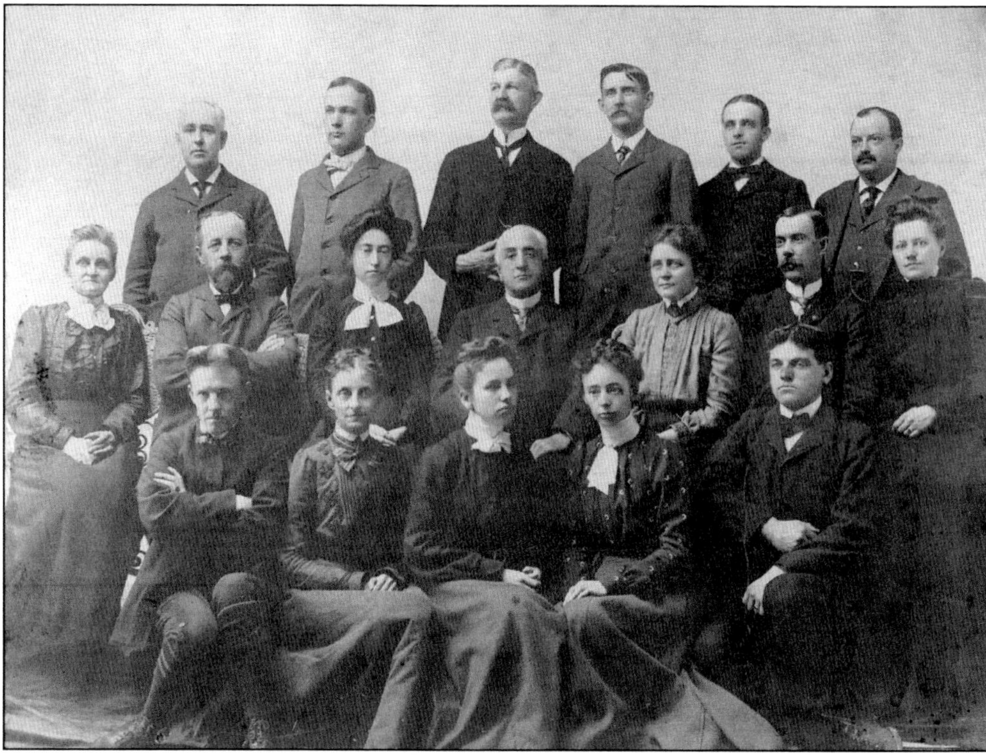

As president of Heywood Brothers and Company when a young man was injured in his factory, Heywood expressed concern that workers and residents must travel to Boston for medical treatment. He had hoped to one day build a hospital in Gardner. He is seen here (second row, center) with a group of his department heads in about 1892. (Courtesy of LHML.)

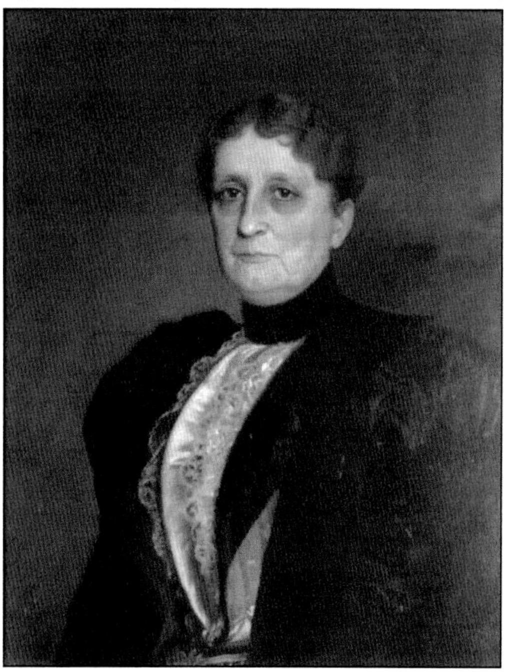

Following Heywood's death, his wife, Martha (pictured), and daughter Helen donated the Henry Heywood Memorial Hospital in memory of their husband and father. This gift to the community included the land, hospital building, and 2,000 shares of the Heywood-Wakefield Company. In addition, the Heywood-Wakefield Company contributed $5,000 to establish a "free bed" fund for the less fortunate.

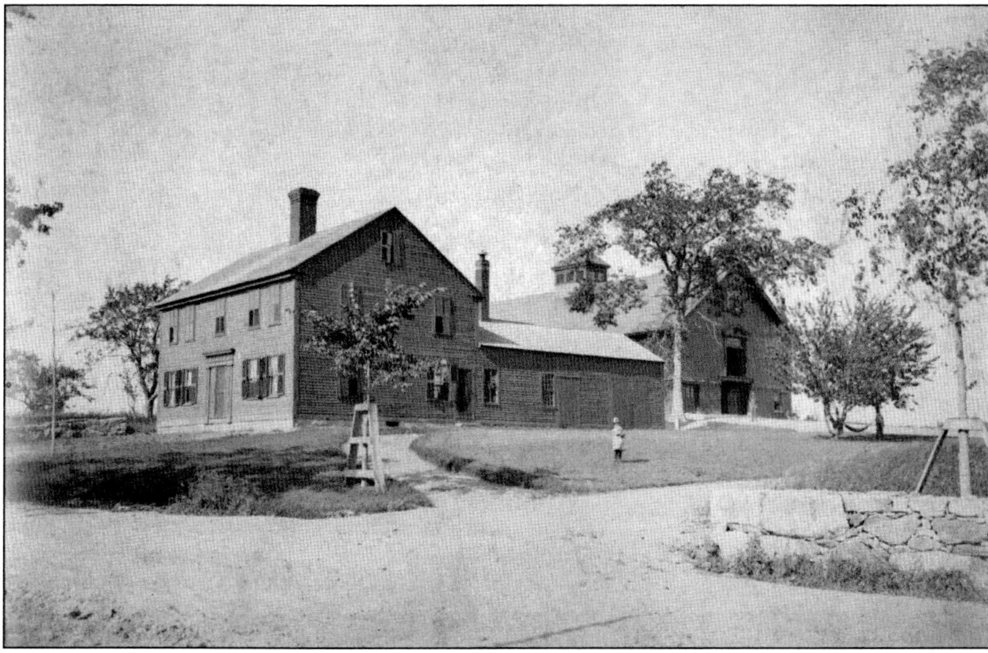

The land currently occupied by Heywood Hospital was originally purchased in the 1770s by Ephraim Temple. It was an operational farm for 150 years and passed down to Martha Temple Heywood. Martha's husband, Henry, invested in further development of the farm and acquired the best livestock available. The Heywood Farm became one of the finest farms in the area. It burned in 1939 in a fire visible from miles away when dry hay combusted in a barn. Today, only the stone ramps to the barn stand on what is now the site of Mount Wachusett Community College. The image above shows the Heywood Farm in the 1890s. Below is an oxen-drawn wagon belonging to the Heywood Farm in the 1920s. Vapor escapes from the oxen's nostrils as ice caused by the cold temperature develops around their mouths. (Both, courtesy of LHML.)

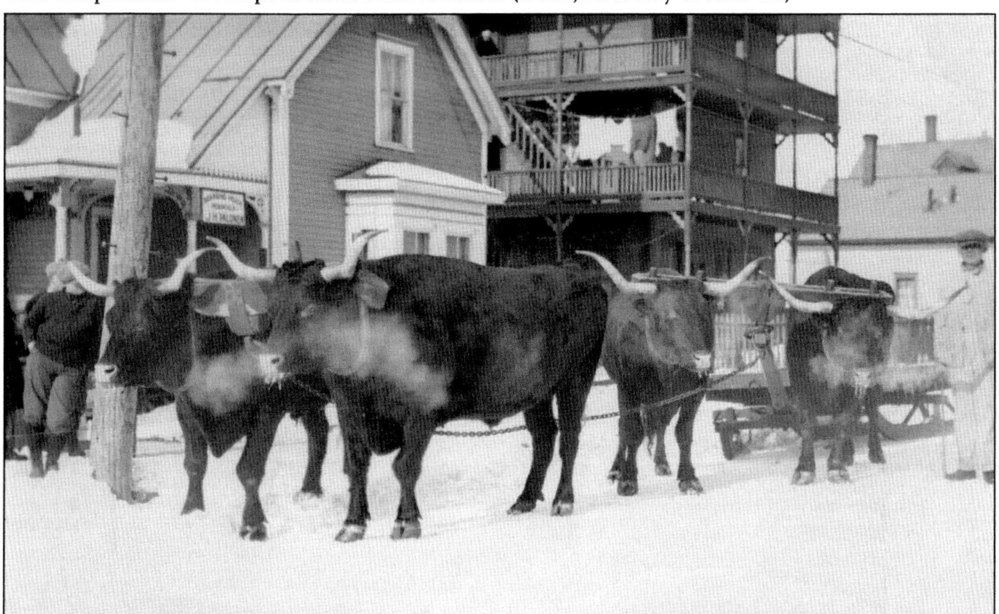

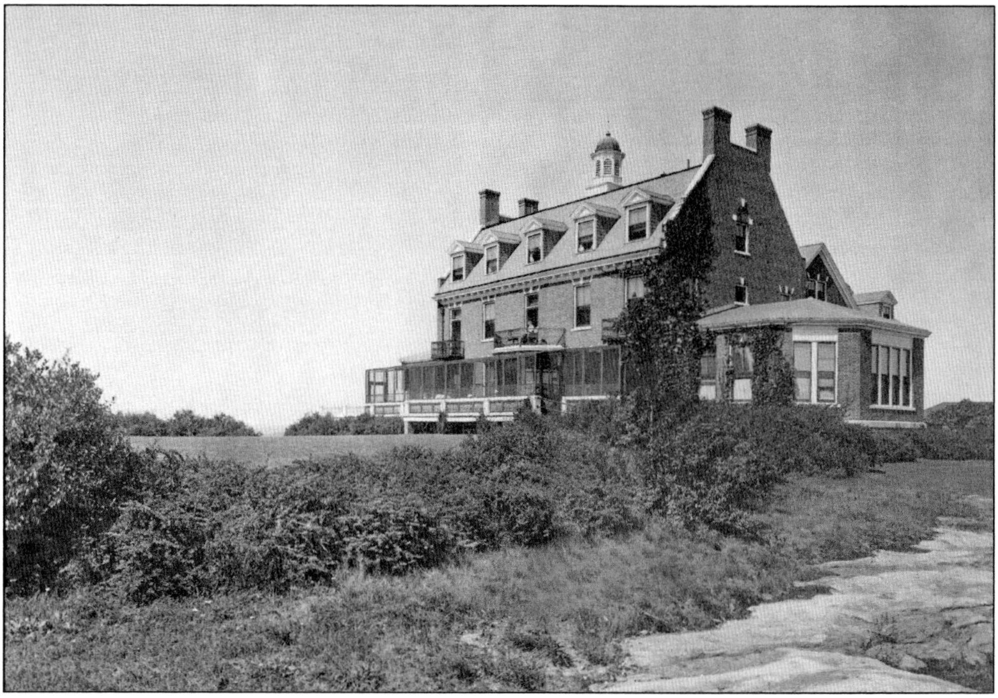

The original hospital was designed by noted Boston architects Kendall, Taylor, and Stevens. A particularly lovely feature was the large solarium facing south with doors that opened to a wide balcony allowing patients to be wheeled out into the fresh air. A formal dedication open to the public was held on June 25, 1907. One account reports an attendance of 1,200 people. After much anticipation, Henry Heywood Memorial Hospital opened its doors to receive patients the following day. Proclaiming it "a magnificent gift," Henry Heywood Memorial Hospital Association's president John D. Edgell's closing words included, "May it forever remain a blessing to this community." Above is a south-side view of the original hospital building in 1907. Below, the hospital sits atop its hill overlooking Crystal Lake with the Gardner Boat Club in the foreground. (Below, courtesy of GM.)

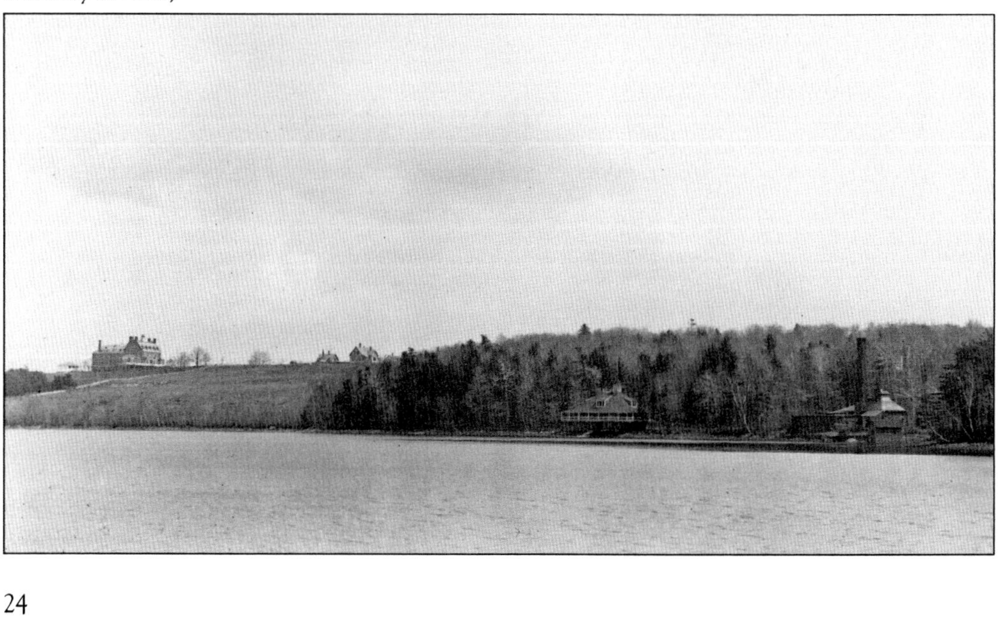

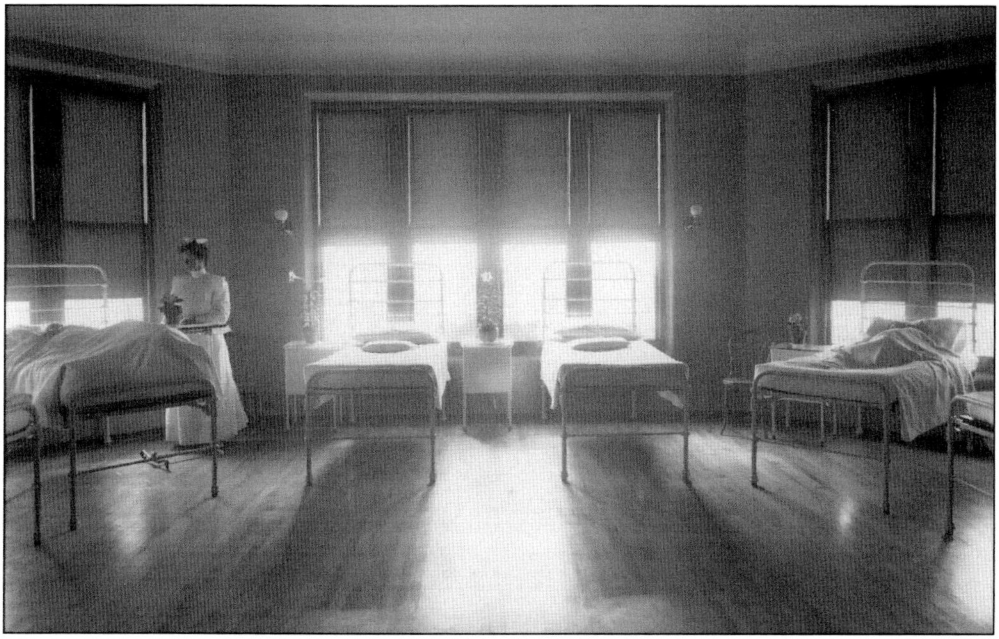

These photographs show the original wards for medical and surgical patients. Located on the first floor were separate but identical eight-bed male and female wards across the hall from each other. Additionally, there were seven private rooms and a maternity ward accommodating six more beds for a total of 29 patients. Plenty of fresh air and sunlight entered the wards via large windows. Besides the attractive fireplaces, there is a distinct lack of equipment around the rooms as opposed to the technology found in a typical hospital room today. Also of note in the photograph below is the patient in cervical traction. The patient is lying with his or her head at the foot of the bed, which has been elevated using blocks. A weight positioned at the end of the bed provides the right amount of "pull."

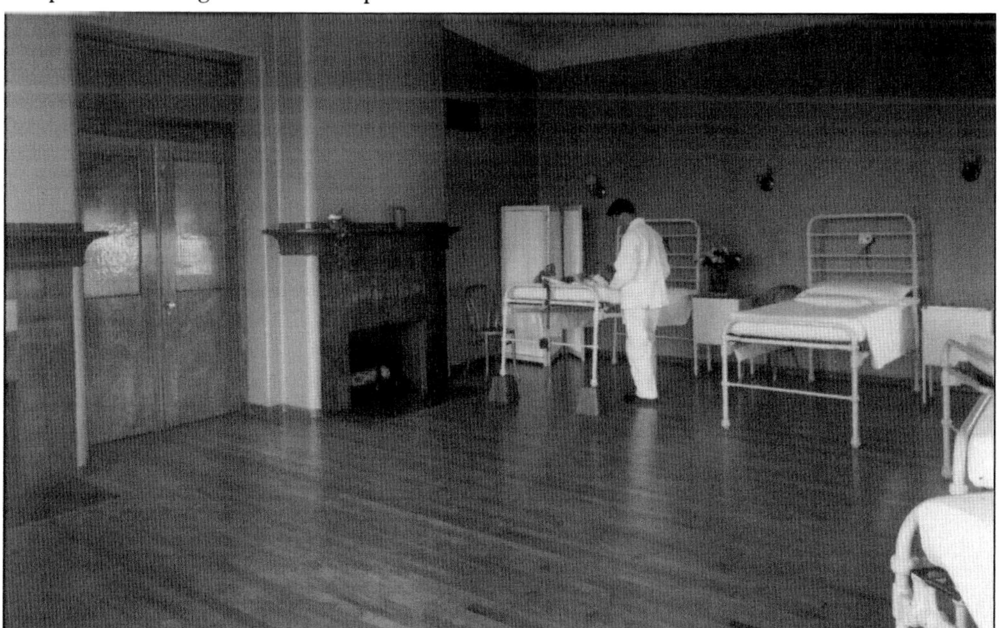

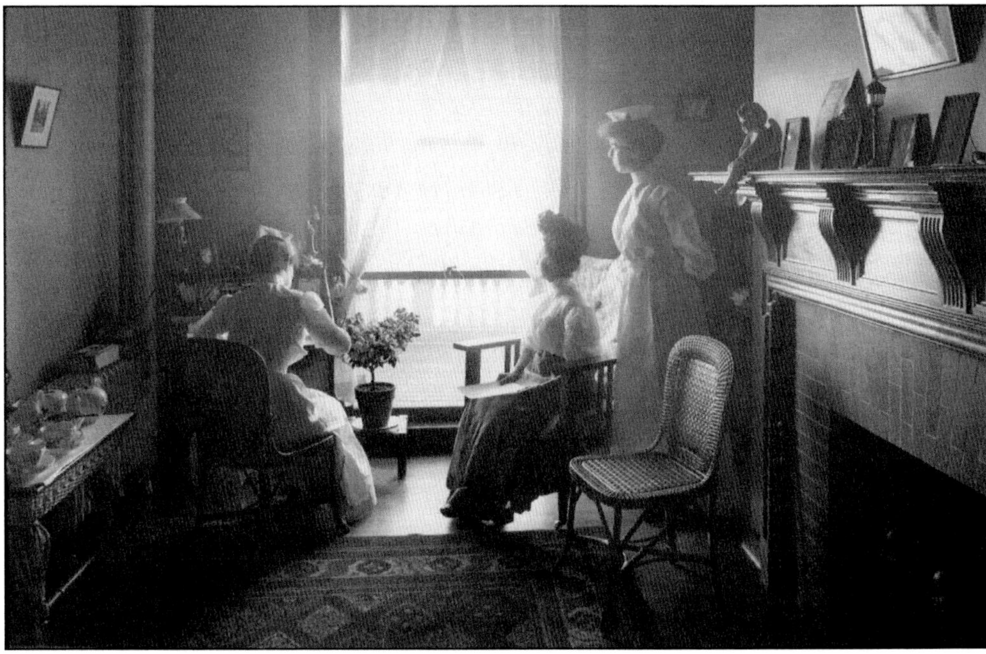

This is the admitting office. The hospital superintendent is recording the information required for an admission while a nurse observes. This location enabled her to look east out the window onto the porch and observe patients as the ambulance brought them into the hospital via stretcher—perhaps the first triage system. The beautiful fireplace and mantel still exist today.

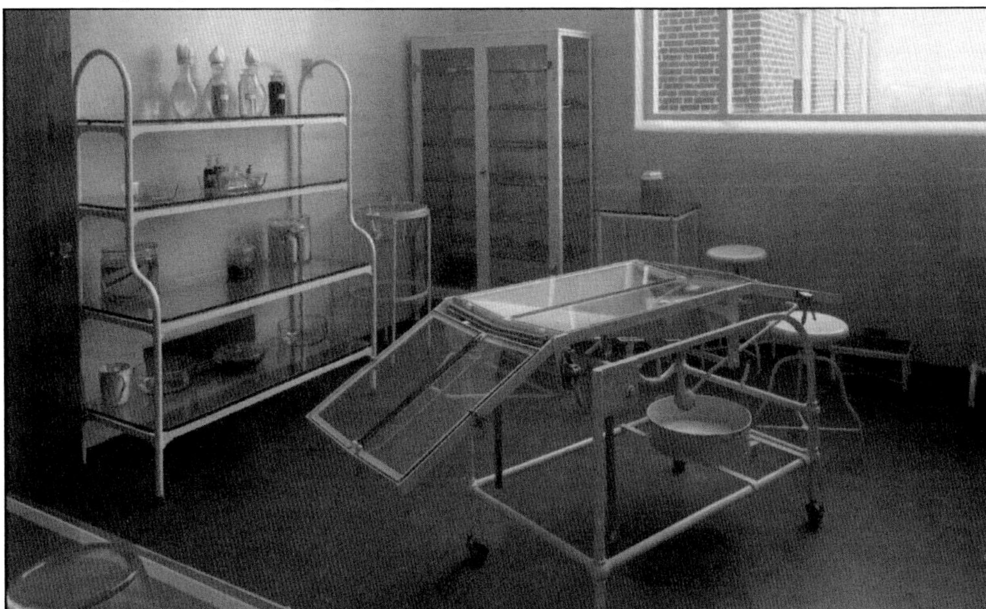

This photograph displays early equipment used in the operating room in 1907 and features the original operating table in the center. Most pieces in the room are made of glass for easy cleaning. Notable is the lack of lamps. Unlike today, only one stationary lamp was provided. The large window shown in the picture purposely faces north to allow sunlight while still allowing the room temperature to remain cool.

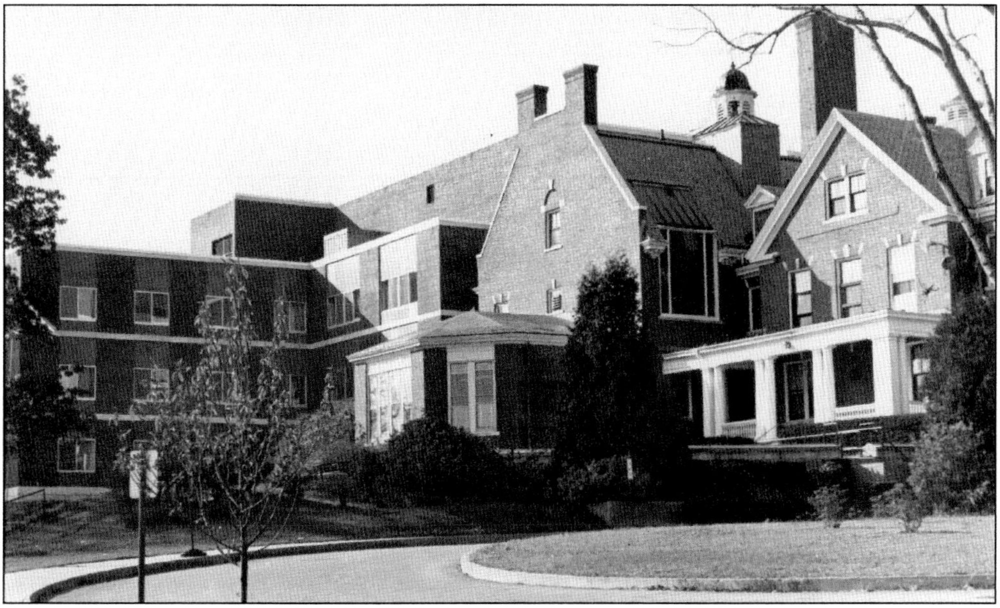

This later view of the hospital building shows the large window in the main operating room facing north just to the left of and above the front porch. This massive window originally stretched up two floors. Although now partially closed off, it is still visible. The image below shows the operating rooms. A second operating room was used for otolaryngology and urological surgery. The floor lamp in this room had a swinging adjustable arm so that it could be focused on the surgical field. It had an extension with a large ball used to swing the lamp about. Dr. Joseph Forte, a retired surgeon, performed surgery in this room and recalls that a nurse would routinely grab the ball of the overhead lamp in this surgical suite, swing it around for repositioning, and inevitably break the windowpane.

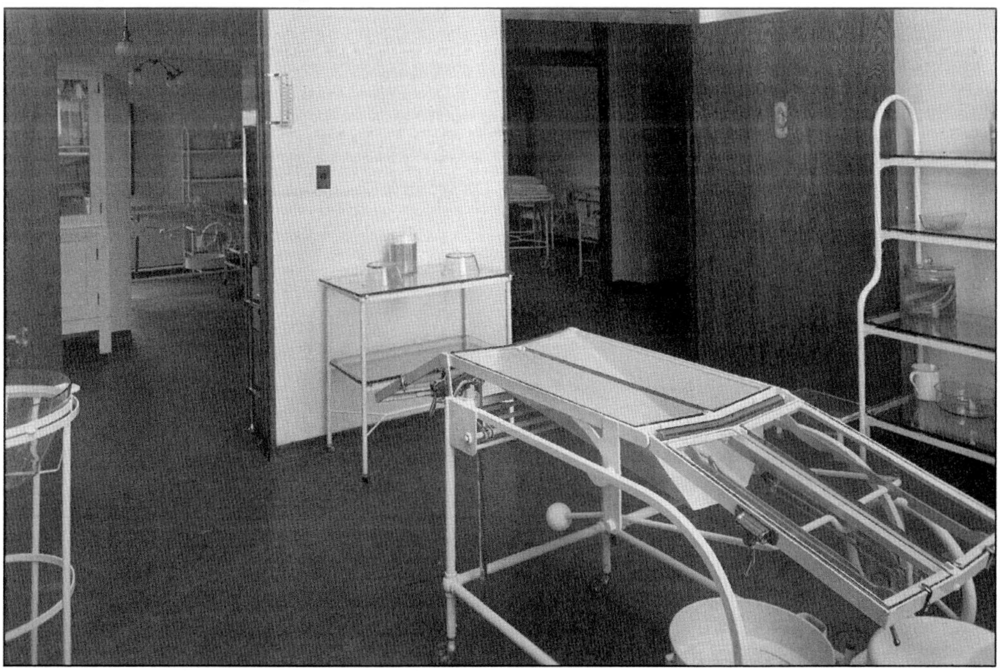

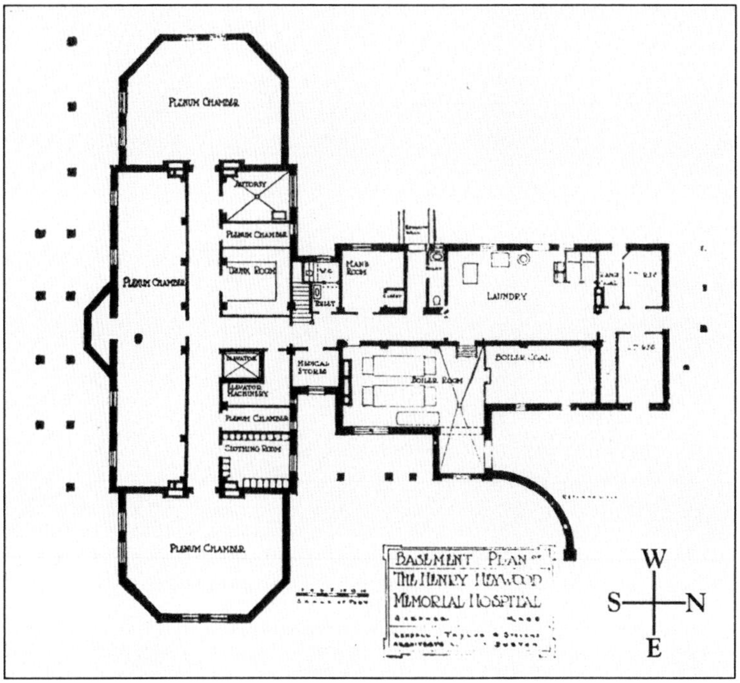

The original building consisted of two principal parts. The southern portion held the patient wards while the northern portion held the administrative and service areas. The basement level had ample space for a boiler room, a coal storage room, laundry facilities, and medical stores. A closer look at this sketch of the basement plan reveals a "drunk room." This room presumably was for patients in need of detoxification.

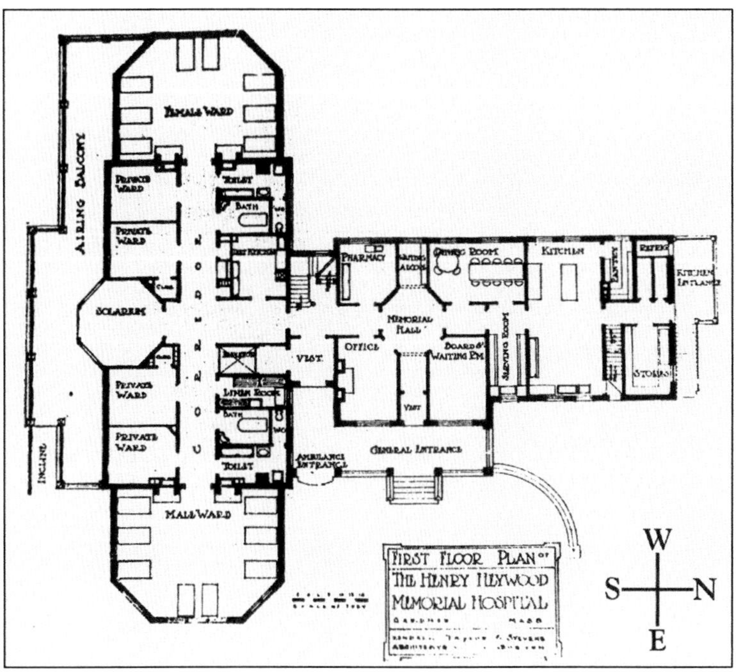

On the first floor of the southern portion were the male and female patient wards, several private rooms, a linen room, bathrooms, and a solarium. Located in the adjacent wing were the main entrance and the ambulance entrance, superintendent's office, boardroom, pharmacy, kitchen and dining room, waiting room, and storage room.

There were two operating rooms located on the second floor of the original building. An electric elevator located by the ambulance entrance on the first floor brought the patients up to the surgical suite and several private rooms. The adjacent wing provided quarters for the matron or superintendent, including a sitting room with fireplace, a bedroom, and private bath. Housing was also provided for the nurses on staff.

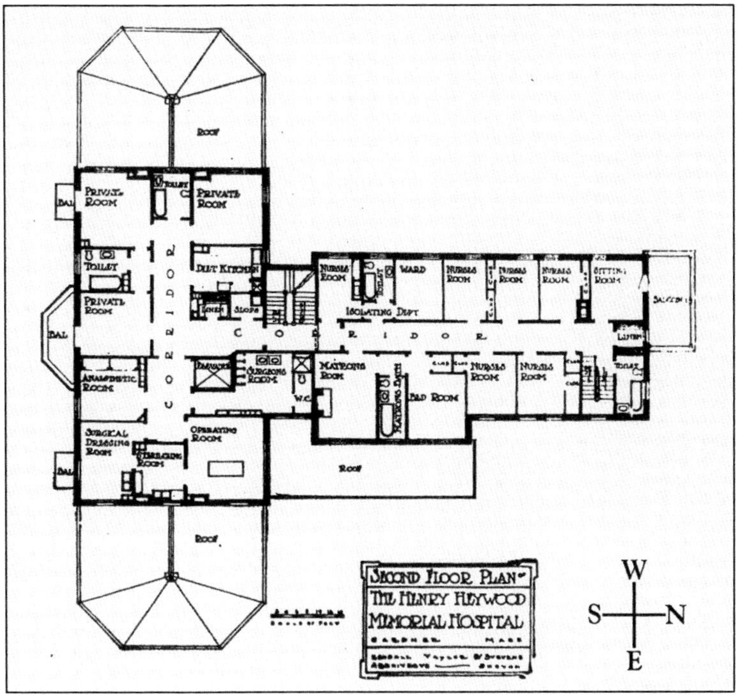

The maternity ward was located on the third floor and consisted of a four-bed ward, two private rooms, a labor room, kitchen, bathroom, and linen room. The adjacent wing consisted of accommodations for nurses and servants. At that time, all the baby linen was washed by the staff nurses.

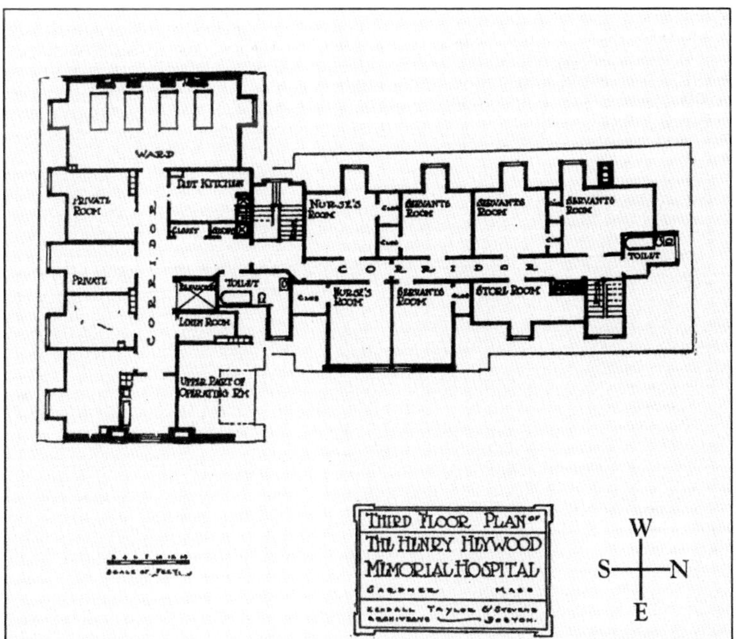

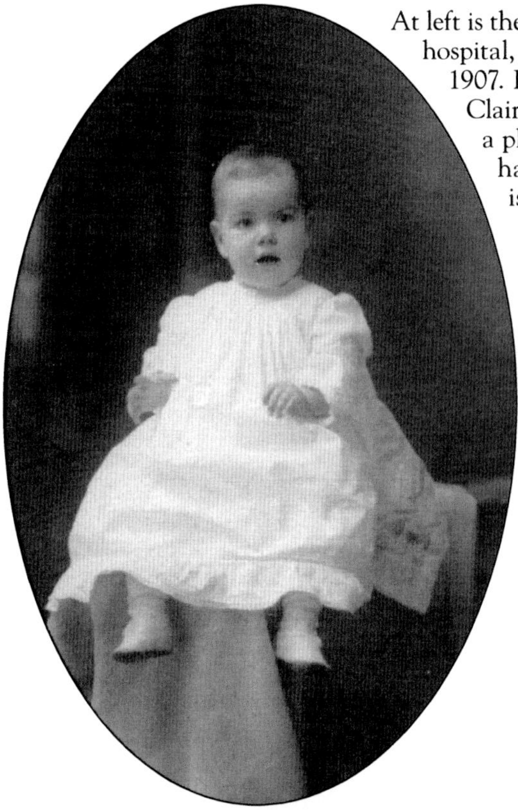

At left is the first baby born at Henry Heywood Memorial hospital, a girl named Elinor Brooks, born on July 5, 1907. Her parents were Edward Adam Brooks and Clair Nichols Brooks. Elinor married Wallace Peck, a photographer from nearby Winchendon. She had no children and died of leukemia. Below is a photograph of a private room. In 1907, a private room cost three times more than a bed on the ward. In addition to complete privacy, amenities included curtained windows, an upholstered chair, and dressers complete with dresser scarves. Rates for residents of Gardner were $7 per week for a ward bed, $21 for a private room, $28 for a private room with bath, or $75 per week for two rooms with a bath.

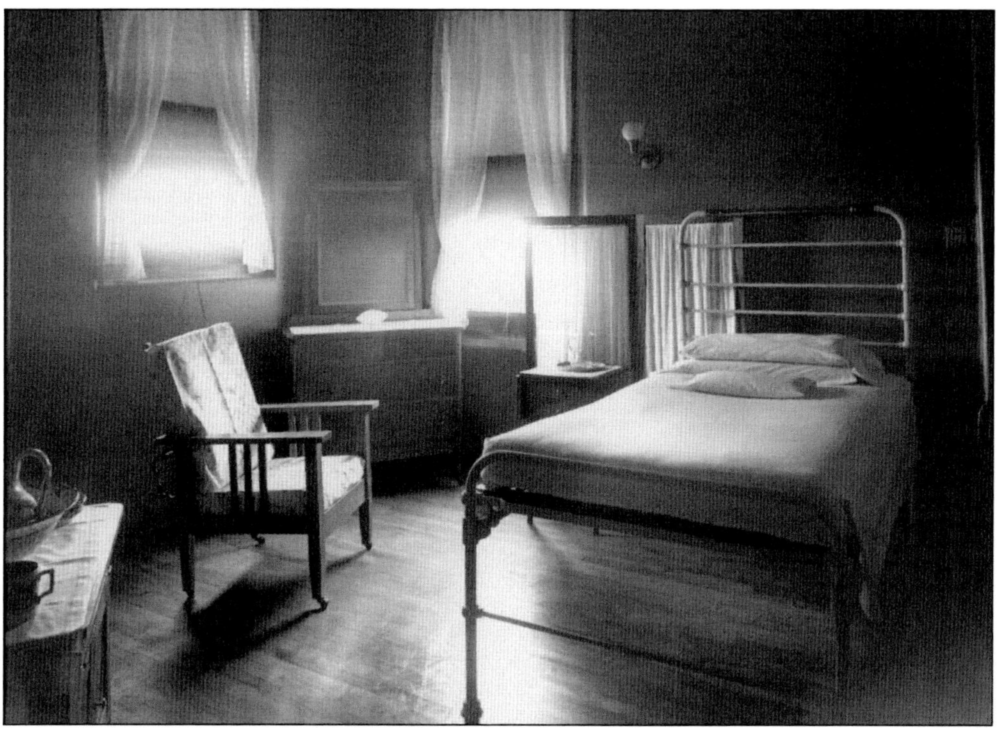

Three

The West Wing and Wartime Expansion

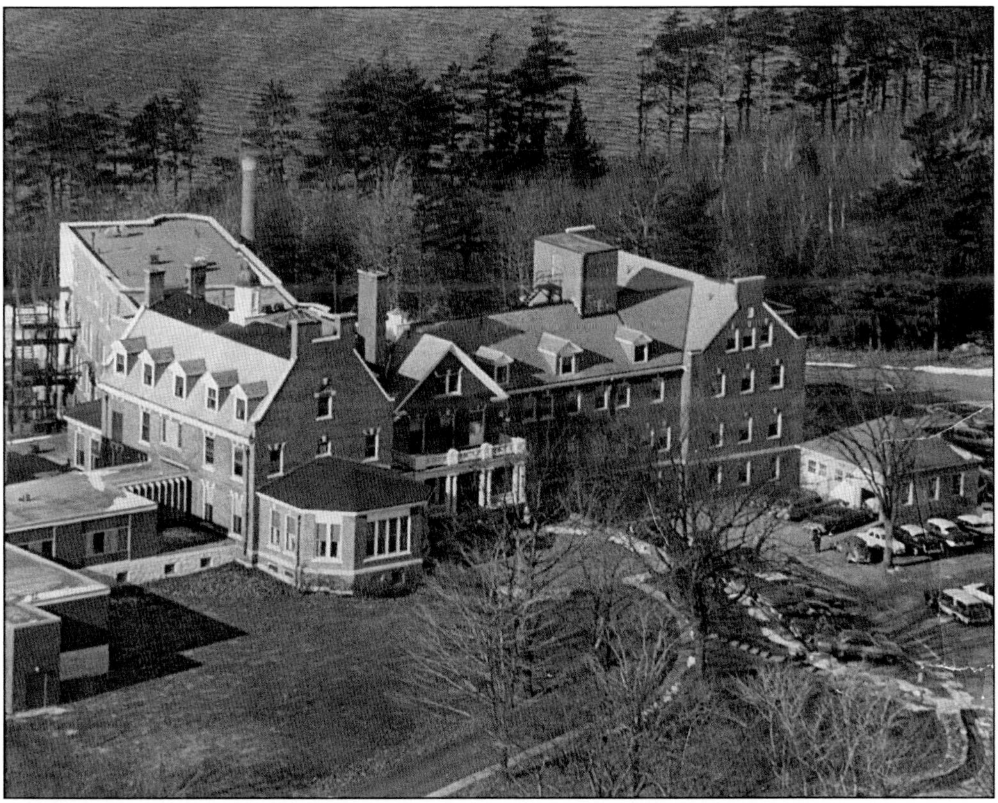

In 1921, Helen Heywood donated the West Wing, seen here with its tall chimney stack to the left rear of the building facing the lake, for maternity and children's care. It was intended to honor her mother, Martha Temple Heywooda. The opening celebration was to be held on October 22, but construction was delayed and Heywood unfortunately passed away prior to the opening of the new wing.

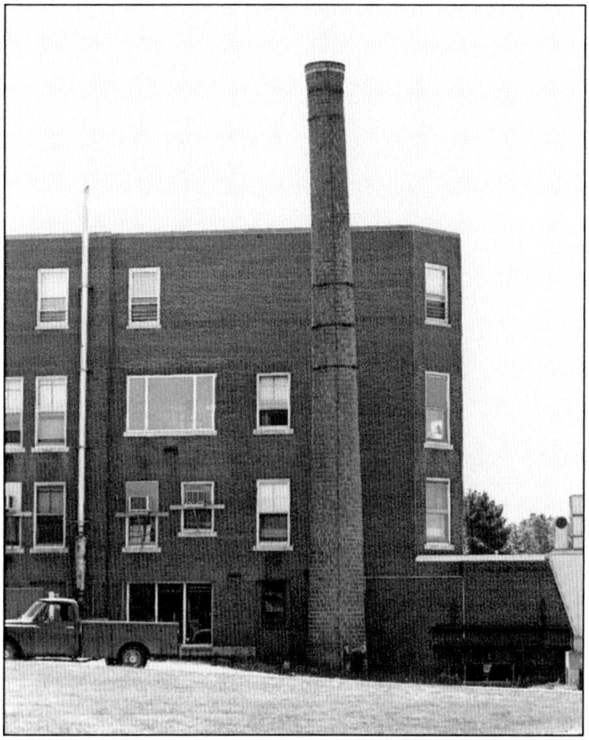

The West Wing was four stories high and rather spacious. It did not have the architectural character of the original hospital building, but it did have attractive bay windows facing west and overlooking Crystal Lake. The wing consisted of a basement and three floors. The basement of the wing housed the boilers for the heating system and various storage areas. Visible in this side view of the West Wing are the four floors, the chimney providing a vent for the boilers, and a partial view of the aforementioned bay windows. The first floor of the West Wing housed a ward for medical and surgical patients. Over the years, this floor became known as the General Floor. In the image below, a nurse is delivering flowers to a patient who has a scenic view of Crystal Lake.

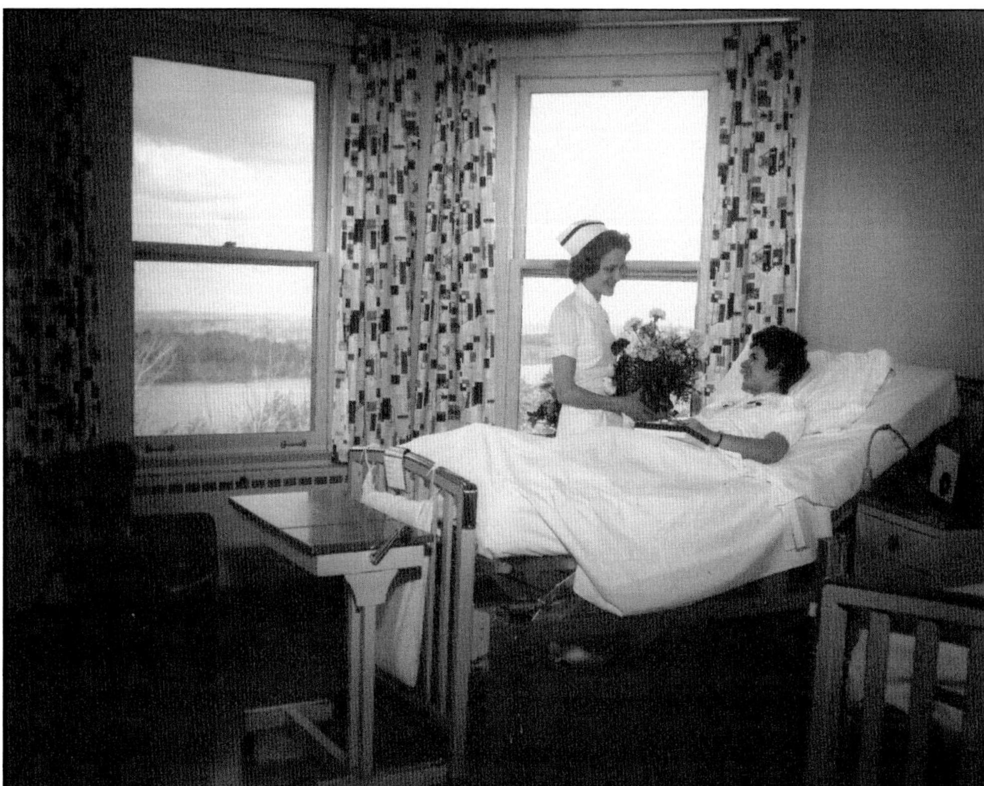

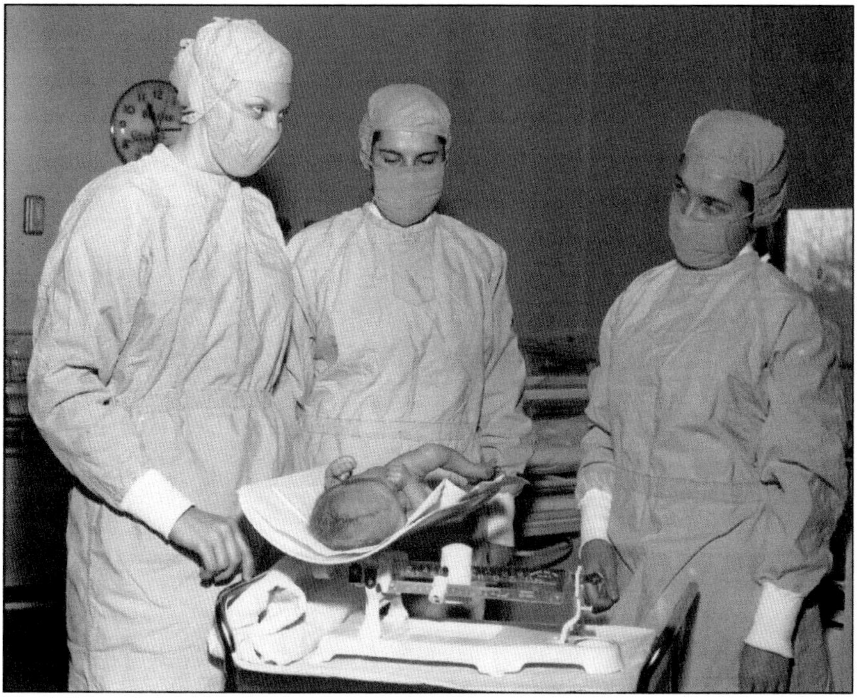

The second floor of the wing housed the maternity ward and the nursery. There was a two-bed labor room and two delivery rooms. The main delivery room was only 16 feet by 17 feet—small by today's standards. It too had a bay window with a beautiful view over the trees to Crystal Lake. The obstetrician undoubtedly enjoyed the view of the lake while waiting, but one wonders if the laboring mother appreciated it. In the image above, a hand-balanced scale is used to weigh an infant. Observing are Henry Heywood Memorial School of Nursing graduate Eunice Dymek and students Georgene Roy and Janyce Charles. The image below shows the nursery with the bassinets all lined up securing their precious cargo. Large wheels on the bassinet holders allow easy transport. The ruffled draperies are not seen in today's nurseries.

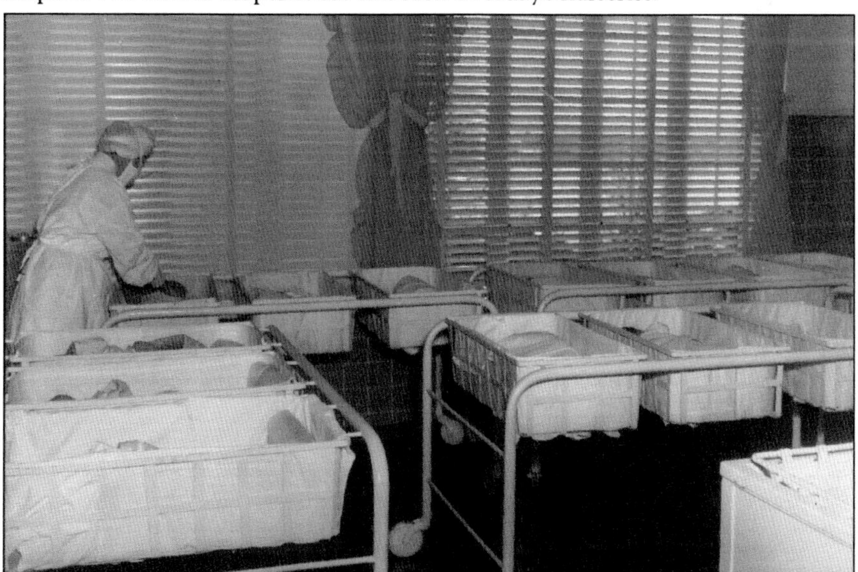

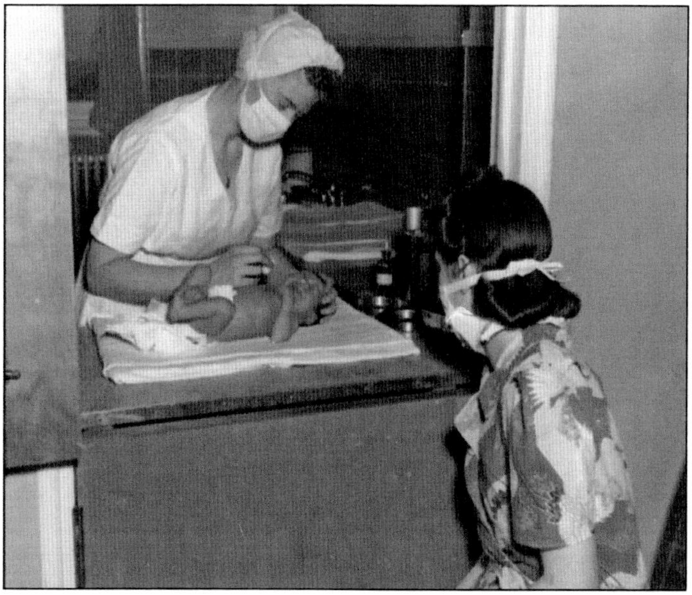

The postpartum rooms consisted of two four-bed wards and two private rooms. Postpartum stays were often a week, compared to the one- or two-day stays of today. The importance of educating mothers in the care of their infants has always been most important. This image depicts a mother's first lesson in bathing her infant.

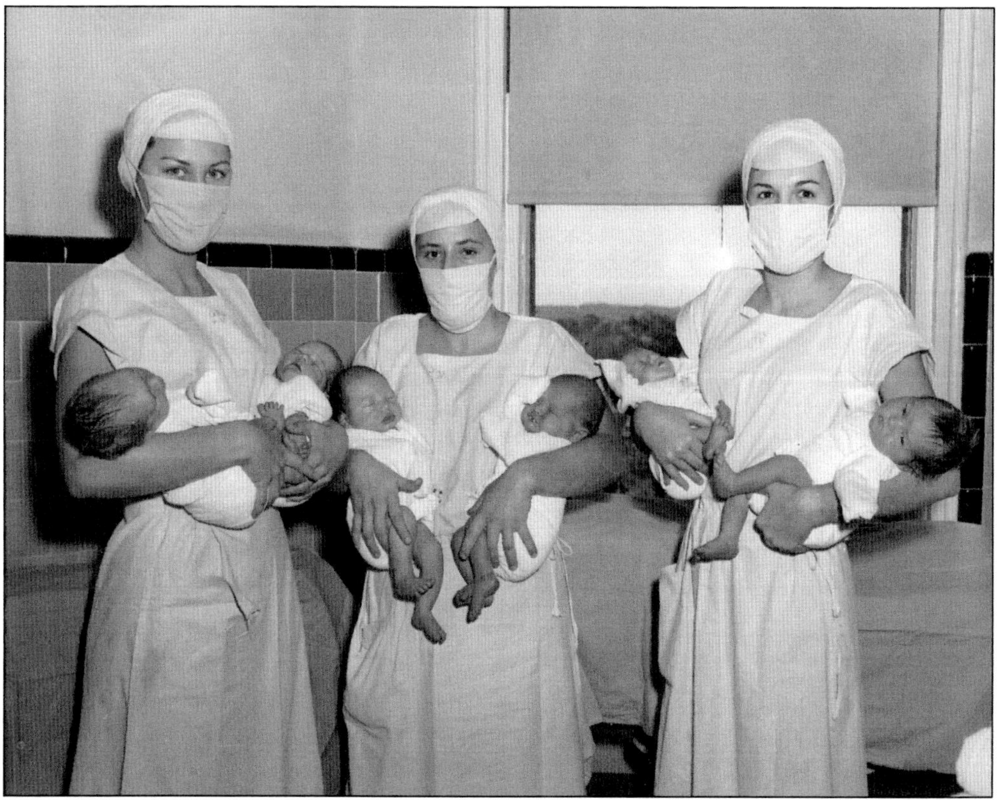

Sets of twins are rare. But to have three sets of twins born and boarding in the hospital at the same time was very unusual. The incidence of twins is approximately one set per 250 births. Since the inception of in vitro fertilization, the rate has increased. The image above from 1954 shows, from left to right, nurses Joyce Austin, Arlene Clouthier, and Jackie Palmer holding the bundles of joy.

The treatment of premature or low-birth-weight infants has been one of the great challenges of pediatrics. Today, infants less than one pound are being saved. However, that was not always true. In the 1930s, it was known that proper warmth and oxygen supply were imperative. This image shows Heywood Hospital's first incubator. The combination oxygen and heater equipment is being tested by registered nurse Aili Taavitsainen (left).

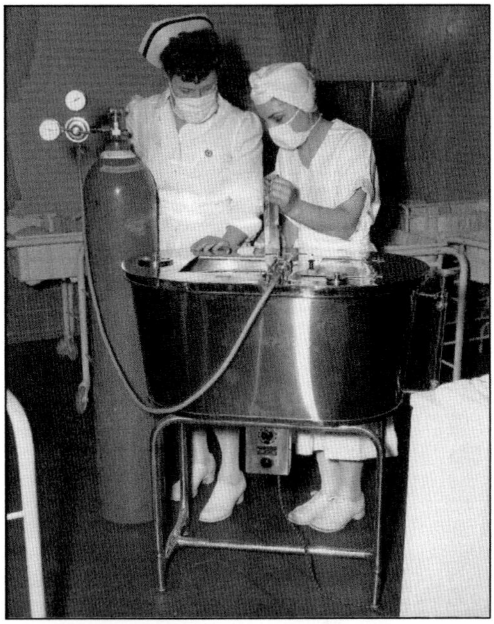

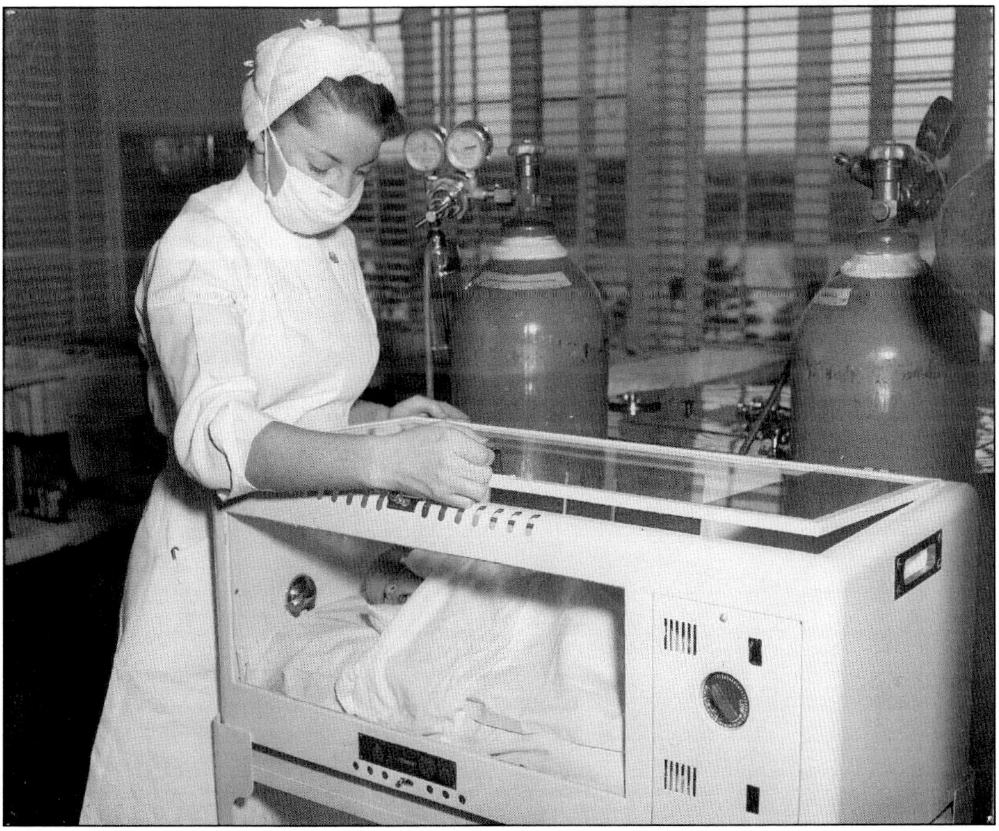

This incubator is a far cry from the early combined oxygen and heat incubator. The infant is very visible through the glass sides and top. This makes observation of breathing patterns and movement much easier. This particular incubator is called a heater crib.

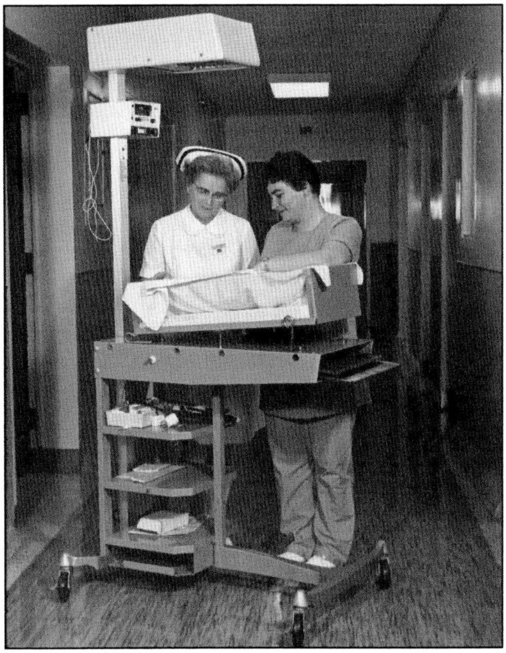

Director of nurses Phyllis Hayes (left) looks over this Jackson heater with registered nurse Jeanne Fitzgerald. Radiant heat is provided from above along with a monitor for vital signs. The unit is mobile and has all of the necessary instruments to intubate an infant and provide intravenous solutions if necessary.

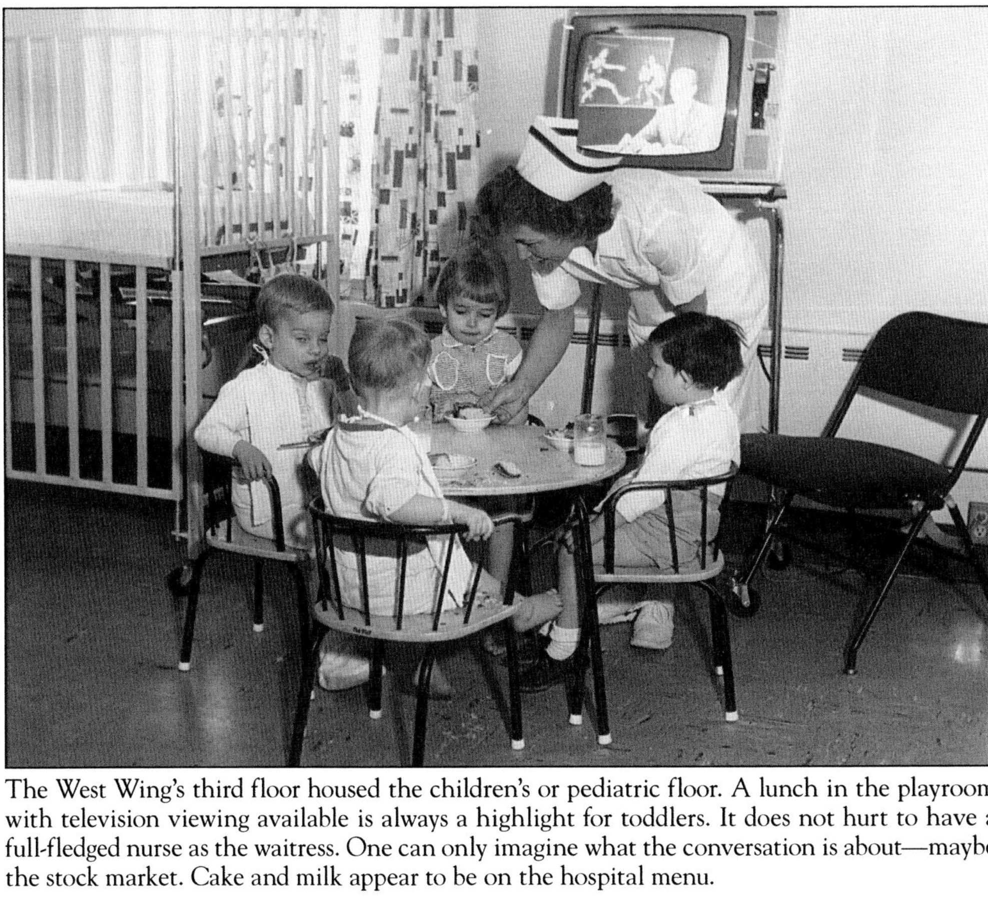

The West Wing's third floor housed the children's or pediatric floor. A lunch in the playroom with television viewing available is always a highlight for toddlers. It does not hurt to have a full-fledged nurse as the waitress. One can only imagine what the conversation is about—maybe the stock market. Cake and milk appear to be on the hospital menu.

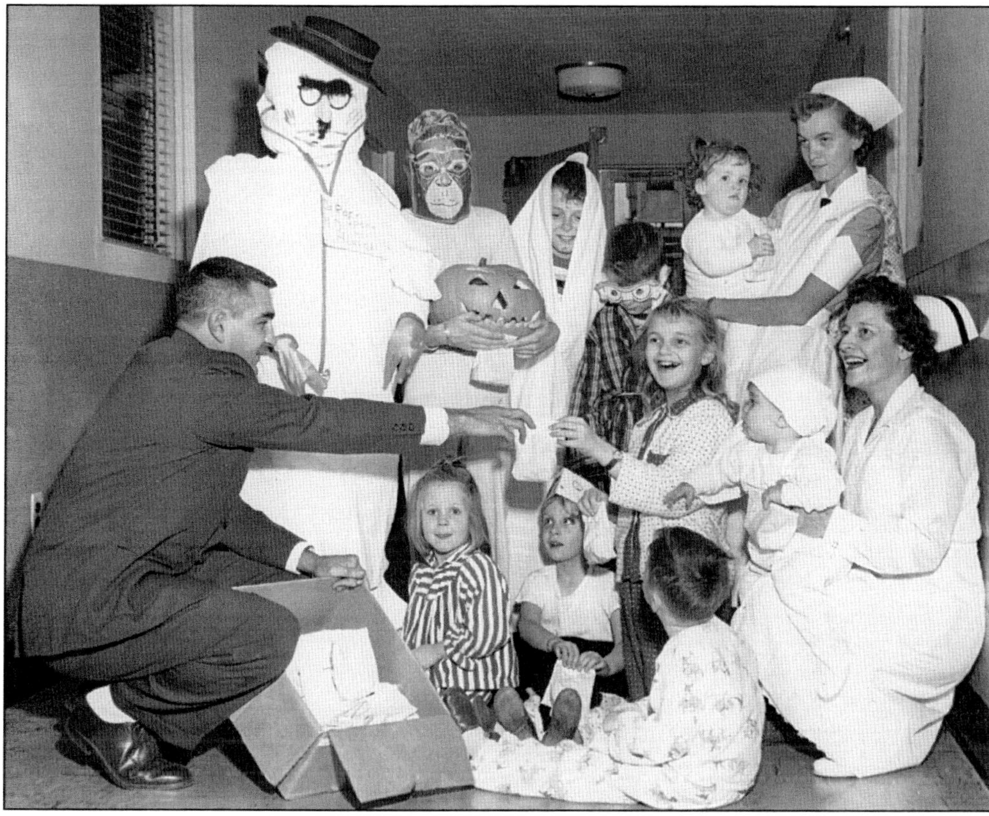

Everyone loves a party—especially a Halloween party. Here, head nurse Anita Dack (lower right) appears to be enjoying the party as much as the children. Raymond LaFontaine, then the recreation director for the city of Gardner, is taking pleasure in handing out goodies. It was not unusual for local organizations to host parties on the pediatric ward.

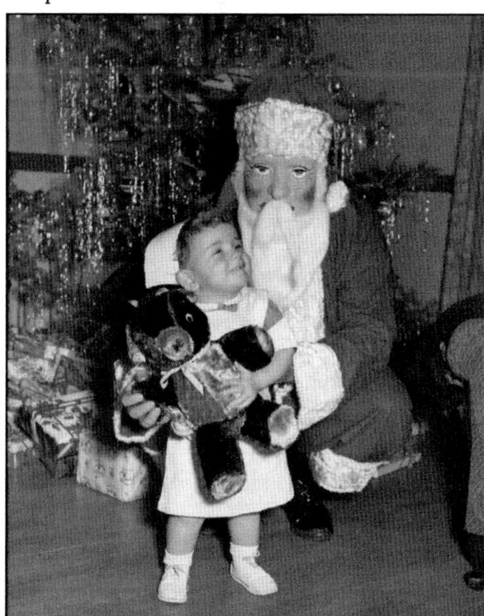

This festive Christmas photograph was taken in 1948. Dressed as Santa is Norman Norcross. The happy little girl is Beverly Lashua, who was a patient at Heywood Hospital for a period of one year. This holiday event was held in the common room in the Nurses' Residence.

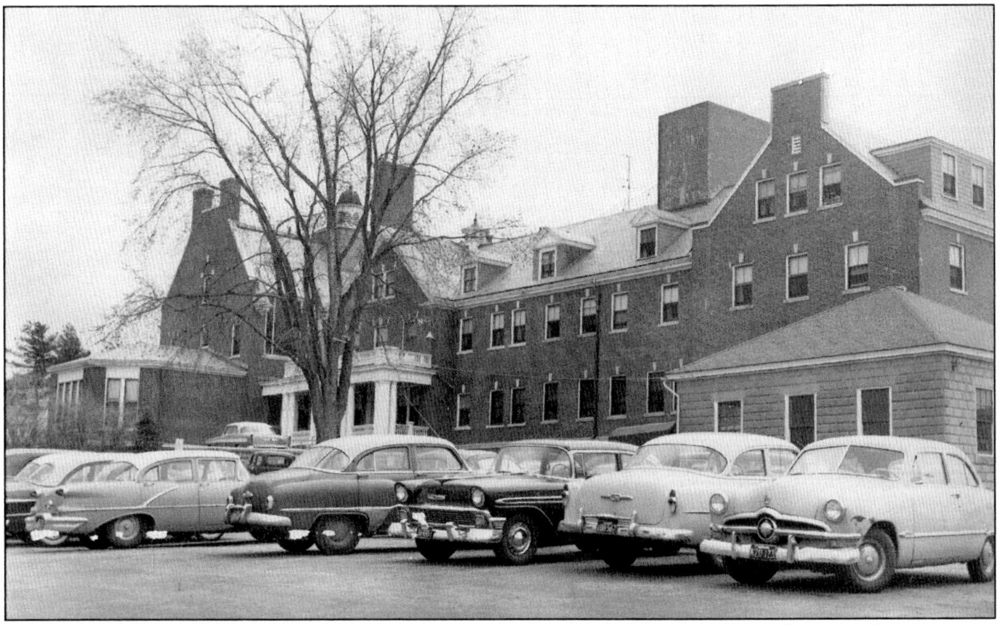

The North Wing of the hospital was built over a period of time during World War II from 1941 to 1945. It was attached to the 1907 building, which housed the original dining hall, administration space, and nurses' quarters. The ground floor housed the kitchen and support services. The first floor provided a new dining room that was often used as the triage area for disaster drills. The second floor was a medical-surgical patient floor that conveniently connected to the 1907 surgical suite. The third floor was a medical-surgical unit considered to be the elite floor because of the single rooms with scenic views. The photograph above shows the completed North Wing in the 1950s. The image below is of the North Wing in the 1970s with the new hospital entrance.

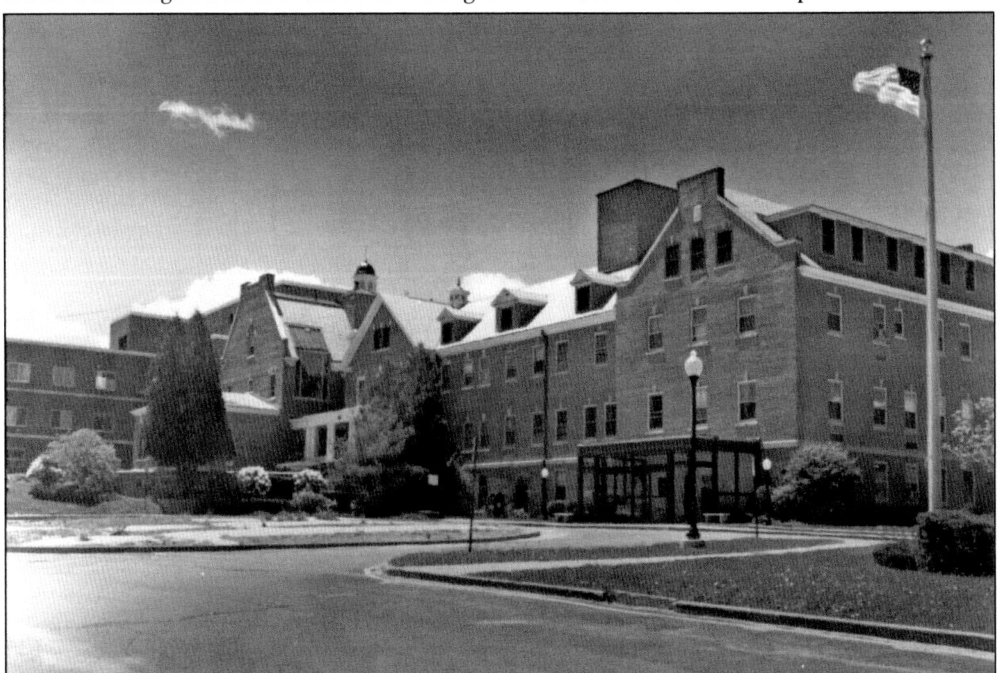

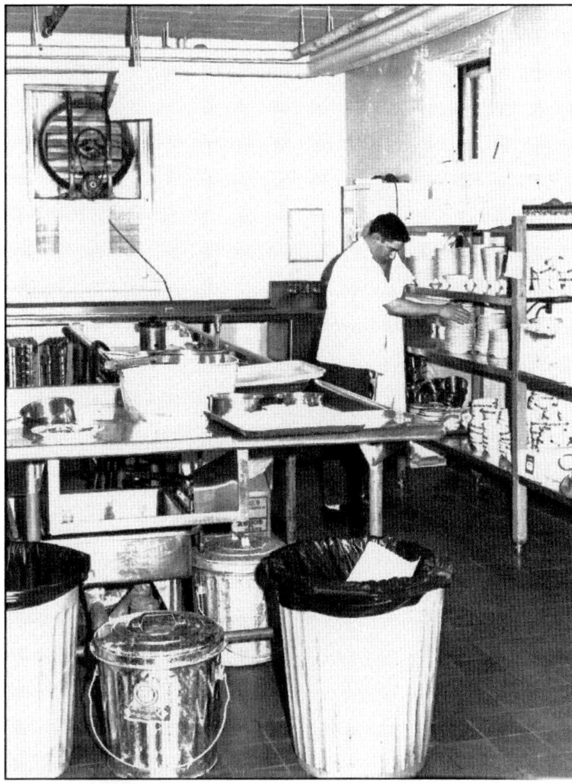

An employee is hard at work in the new kitchen. John Debasitis, employee of 42 years, is one of three generations that has worked for the hospital's food service and remembers the laborious biweekly chore of removing and cleaning the window fan seen in the upper left. The covered metal cans in the foreground are used to collect food scraps for the pigs of the local farmer who picked up the scraps daily in his old truck. Below is the information desk and switchboard operator. Today's switchboard operator is surrounded with state-of-the-art technology. Incidentally, a report from the director of Henry Heywood Memorial School of Nursing in 1941 states, "The new addition [North Wing] to the hospital has already proved its value in the conservation of nursing service. The nurses' dining room is commodious, attractive, and the atmosphere restful."

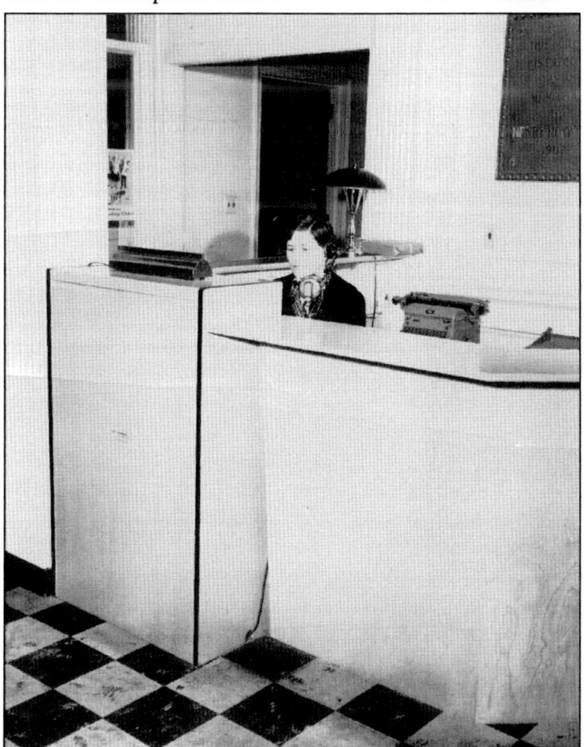

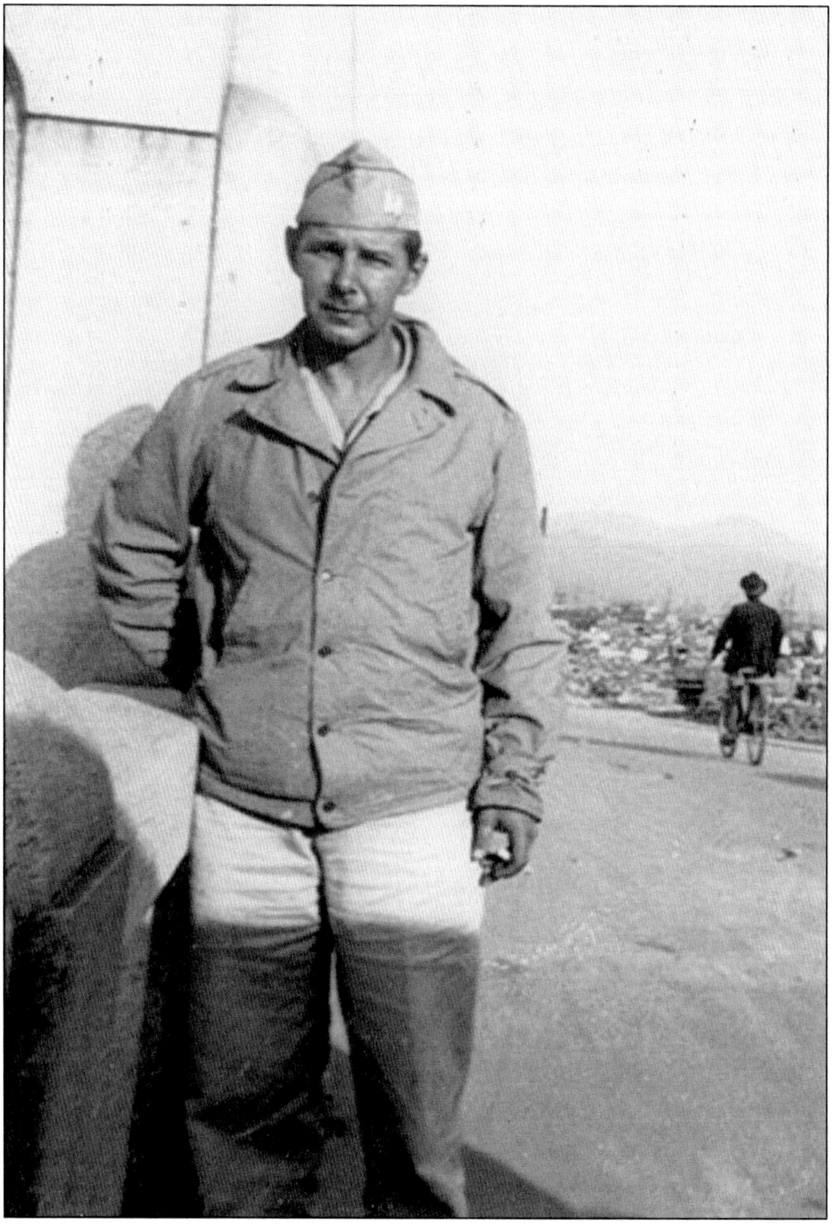

During World War II, Dr. Keijo K. Jolma was one of many Heywood Hospital physicians who served their country. A surgeon in the US Army, he treated the first wounded during the invasion of the Philippines. It was there that he treated the "first human bomb." Jackie Miles was standing beside a palm tree when he was hit in the chest by a 20-millimeter shell from a Japanese airplane. The shell failed to explode. Jolma was one of the physicians who removed the live shell from his chest. Miles lived to marry his childhood sweetheart in 1945 and father seven children. Jolma served the people of Gardner for 24 years until his death at age 52. Here is Jolma in Hiroshima following the dropping of the atomic bomb. In a letter to his wife, he writes, "The damage caused by that one bomb is indescribable . . . I talked to three Japanese who were among the few survivors and they all said that it was like a flash of lightning and wind, but they heard no explosion." (Courtesy of Peter Jolma.)

Four

Henry Heywood Memorial Hospital School of Nursing

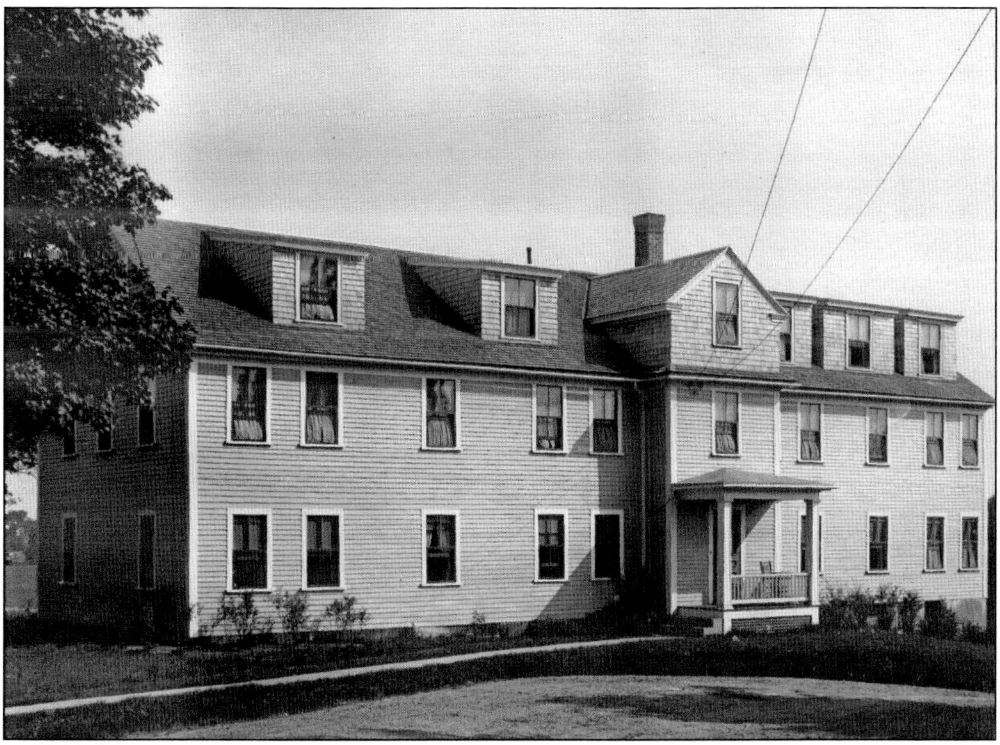

In 1908, Helen Heywood donated a large farmhouse to Henry Heywood Memorial Hospital, which was located directly across the street. From 1926 through 1970, this three-story building was home to the Henry Heywood Memorial School of Nursing, doubling as the residence for the students. Additions were made as the school expanded. After the school closed, it became an administration building for the hospital. This photograph predates any additions.

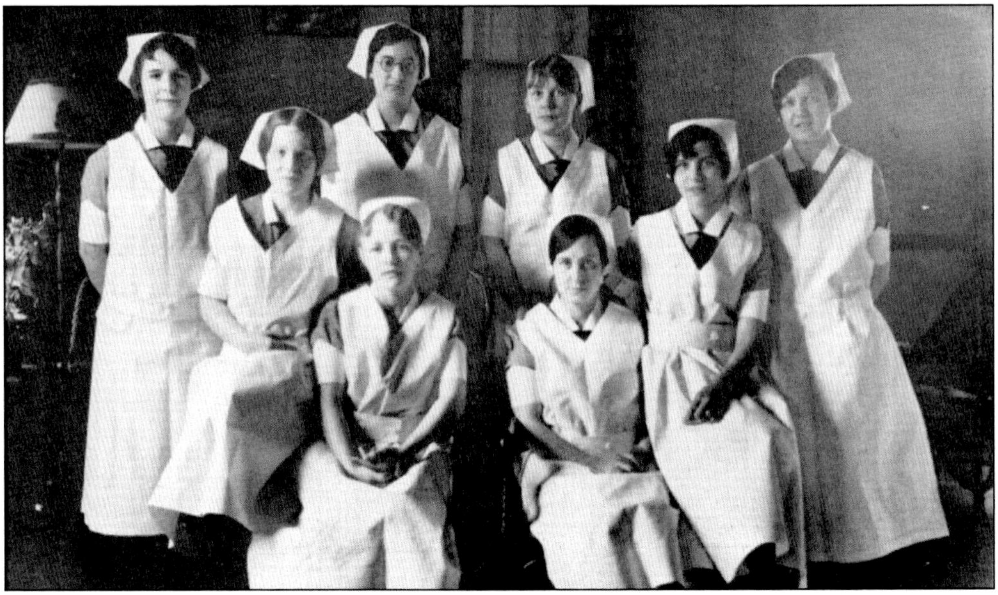

The nursing school's principal was Beatrice K. Barnes, 1921 graduate of the Army School of Nursing. The graduating ceremony for the first class of nursing students was held on October 24, 1929—just five days before the great stock market crash of 1929. Pictured here are Grace Doherty Holmstrom, Elizabeth Gale Furbush, Vieno Janhonen Northridge, Mae Kroczur Smith, Frances Petrowski Suominen, Ingrid Poikonen, Mildred Shepard Kay, and Laura Williams Murdock.

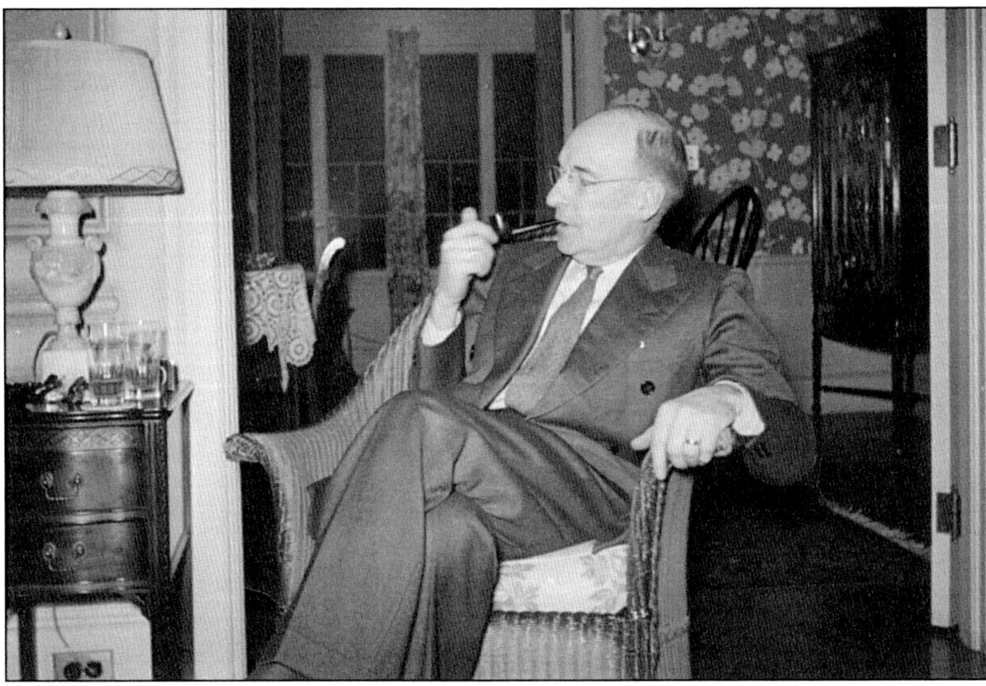

Dr. Charles E. Thompson was the superintendent at the Gardner State Hospital for most of 1902 through 1949. Thompson instituted the first accredited school in the country for licensed attendants. His credentials made him quite fitted to the position of chairman of the Training School Committee, the governing board that oversaw the nursing school's activities.

As chairman of the Training School Committee, Dr. Thompson presided over the first capping ceremony. Students successfully completing the three-year program that stressed basic nursing science as well as clinical training were honored. The photograph below depicts a capping ceremony for graduating nursing students from the class of 1949. The woman at left is dressed as Florence Nightingale and is holding the "lamp of knowledge," as was the tradition. Each graduate also holds a candlelit lamp as they are capped. Graduates all take the Nightingale Pledge. The nursing arts instructor capping the graduate is Marjorie May. Local radio station WHOB, now WGAW, is present to broadcast the momentous event.

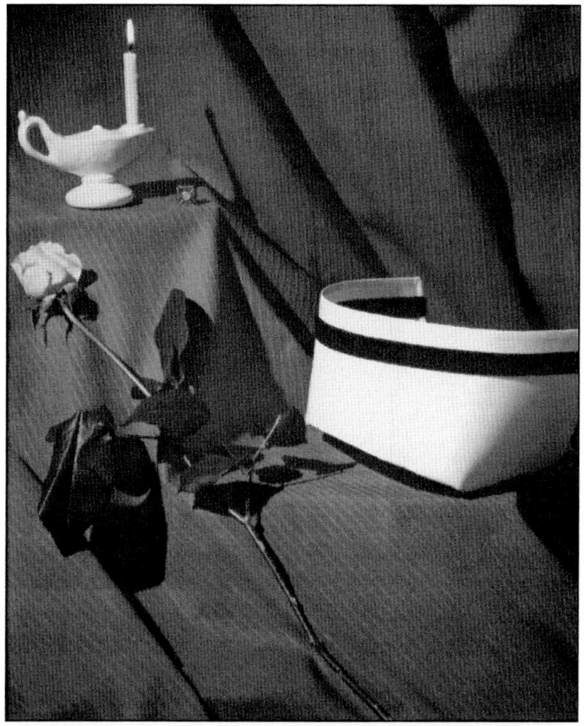

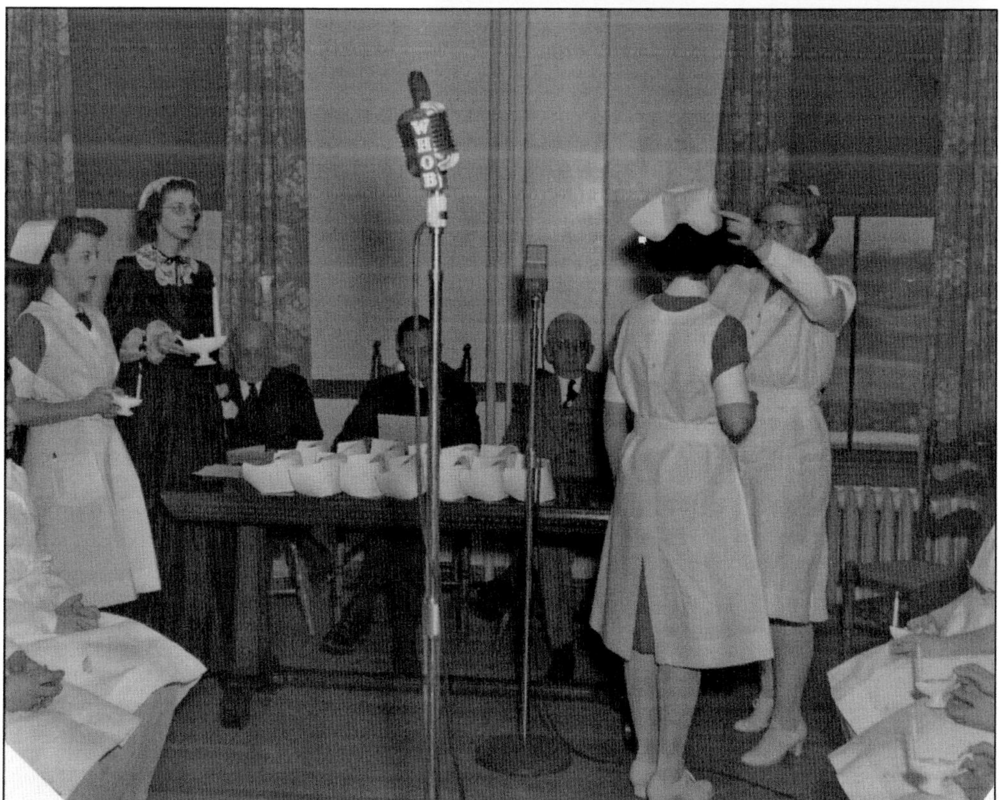

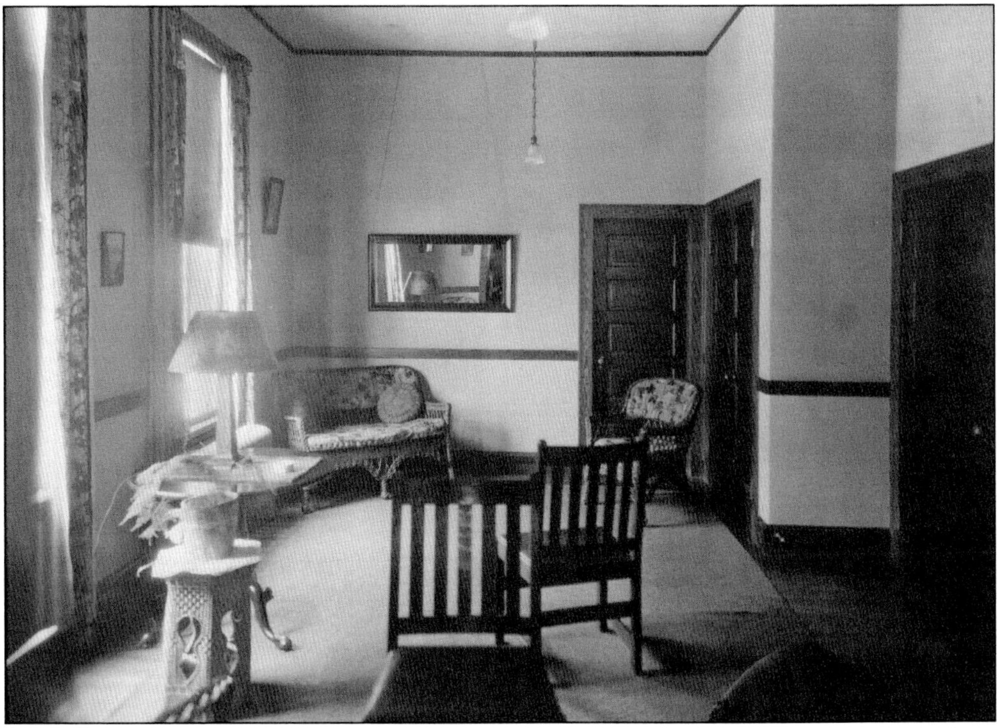

All residential rooms in the Nurses' Residence were attractively furnished single rooms. Bathing facilities were described as adequate. On the first floor, there was a large reception room, or common room, and two small sitting rooms that were often used for studying, informal gatherings, and holiday entertaining. A lecture room with chairs for 18 was also located on the first floor. Dining facilities for the students were on the first floor of the hospital building across the street. Referred to as the East Sitting Room, the space shown above was located just to the right after entering the building. The furniture was most likely manufactured by the Heywood-Wakefield Company. Below, two students study together in one of their bedrooms in 1947.

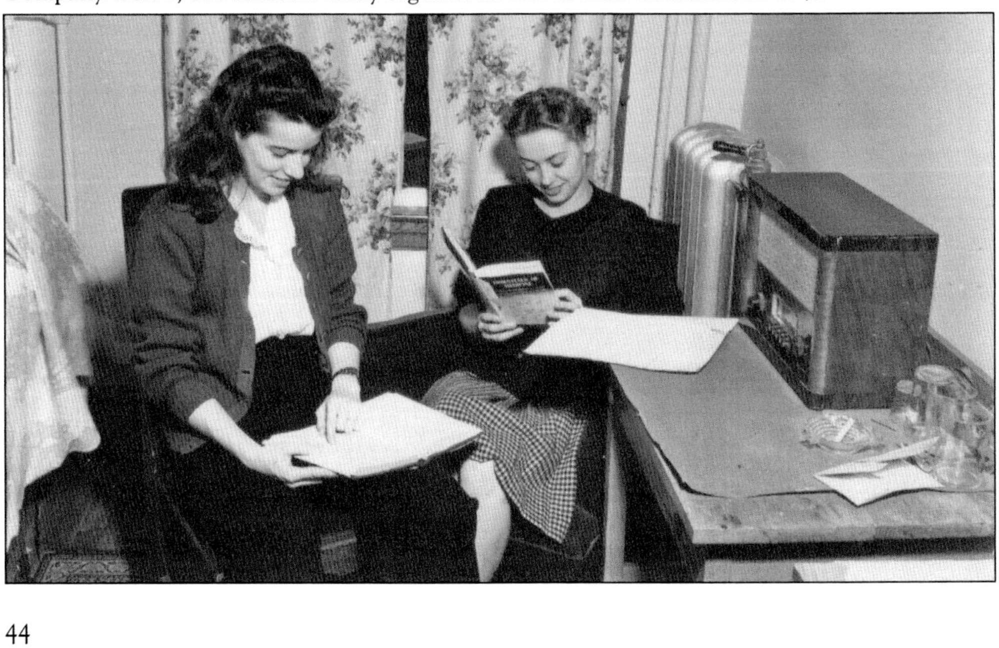

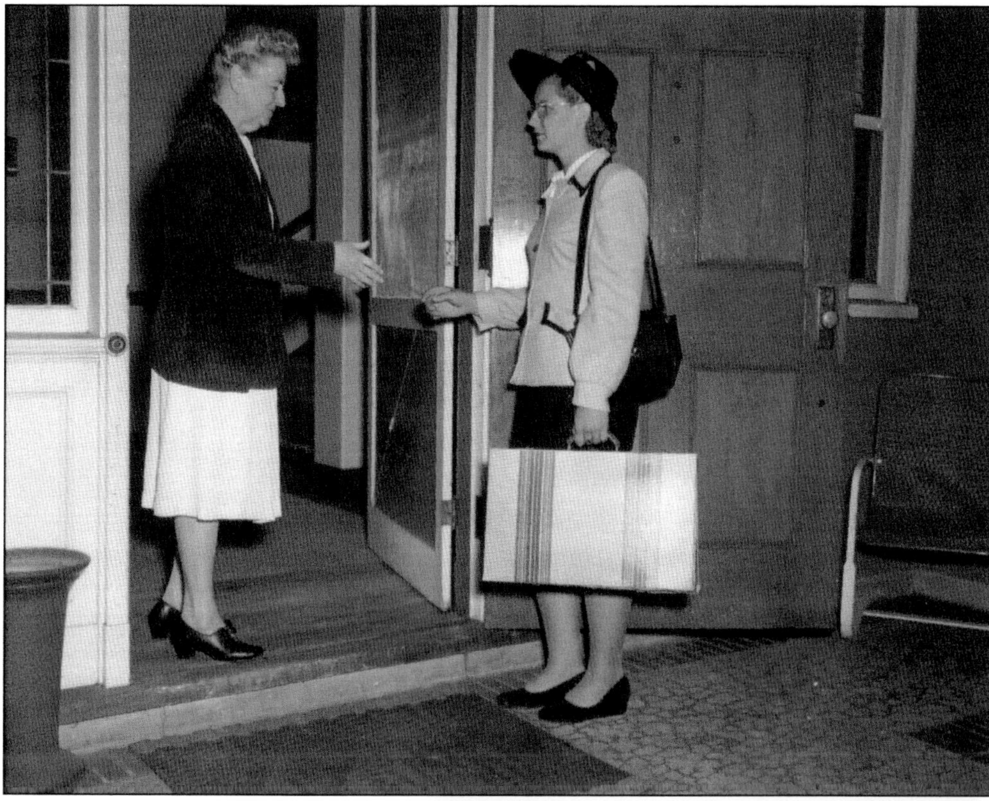

A housemother was in residence to welcome new students, as seen here in September 1947. Another important job of the housemother was to oversee behavior. According to one 1957 graduate of the school, rigid rules were in place, as it was felt that if the students were to one day be responsible for the lives of patients, they needed to be of good character. Despite this, she does recall some of her classmates using the fire escapes to sneak out at night. The bedroom at right belonged to the housemother or nursing instructor. Again, the furniture is recognizable as manufactured by the Heywood-Wakefield Company. The Hospital Aid Association generously furnished all of the bedrooms in the Nurses' Residence.

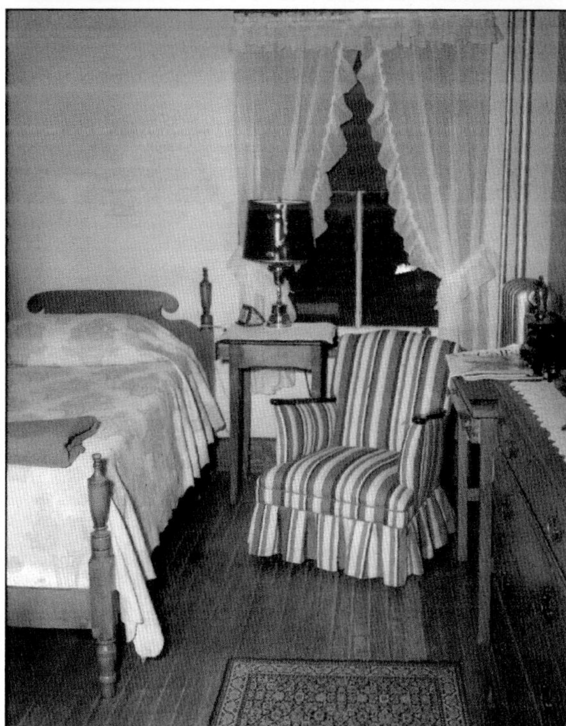

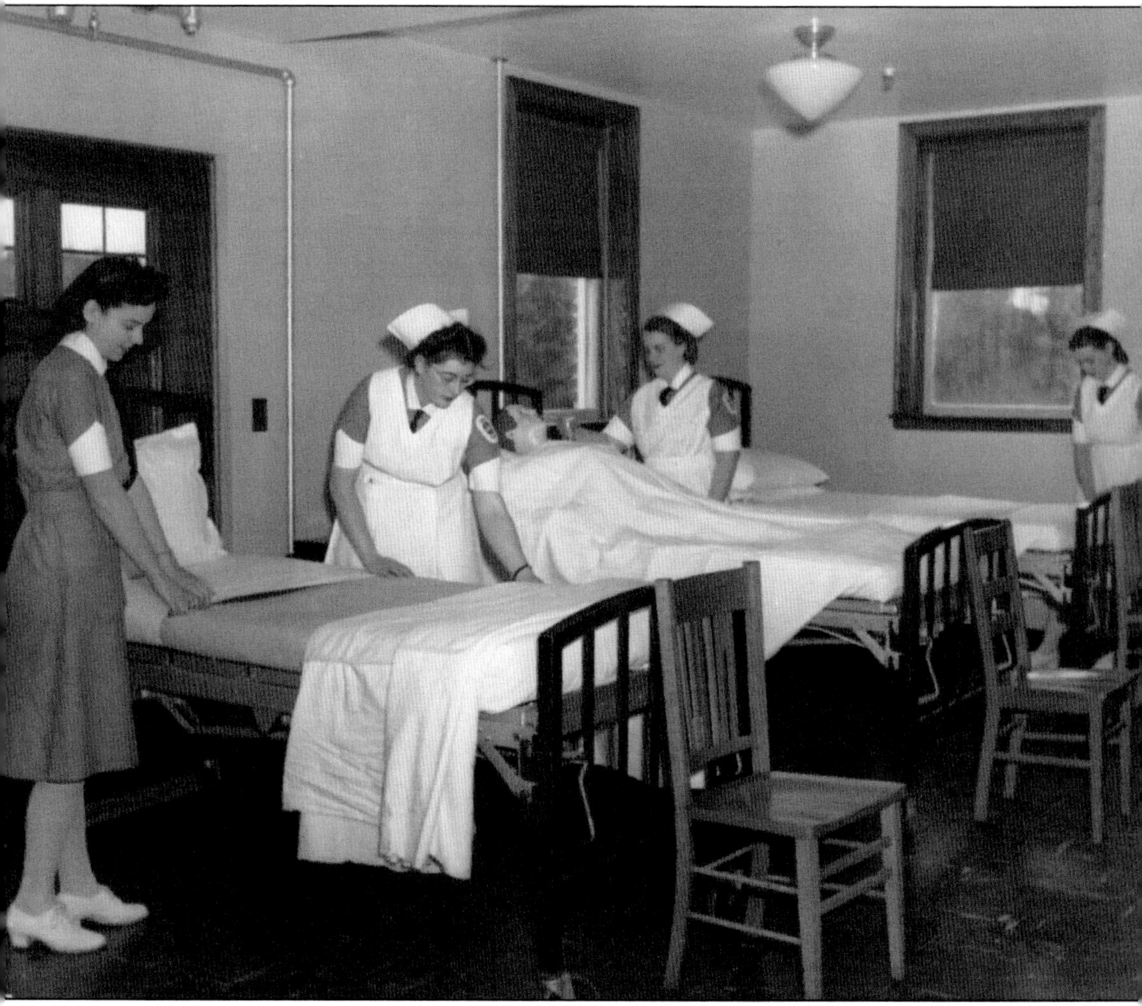

In 1937, a typical day in the life of a first-year student nurse began early with breakfast and tidying her room. Classes began at 7:30 a.m. with the theory and practice of nursing followed by instruction in anatomy and physiology. Most days were free for lunch and recreation from 11:30 a.m. to 1:30 p.m. Classes in ethics, chemistry, hygiene, and sanitation resumed for the remainder of the afternoon. Members of the medical staff provided some of the class instruction. These students are receiving instruction in a nursing arts class in 1945. The nursing arts laboratory was in the basement level of the Nurses' Residence. This class taught skills such as how to properly make a bed, take a patient's blood pressure, and safely provide a drink of water to a patient. The student at far right is making a "closed bed." The two students at left are making an "open bed"—a bed that is ready for a patient to occupy.

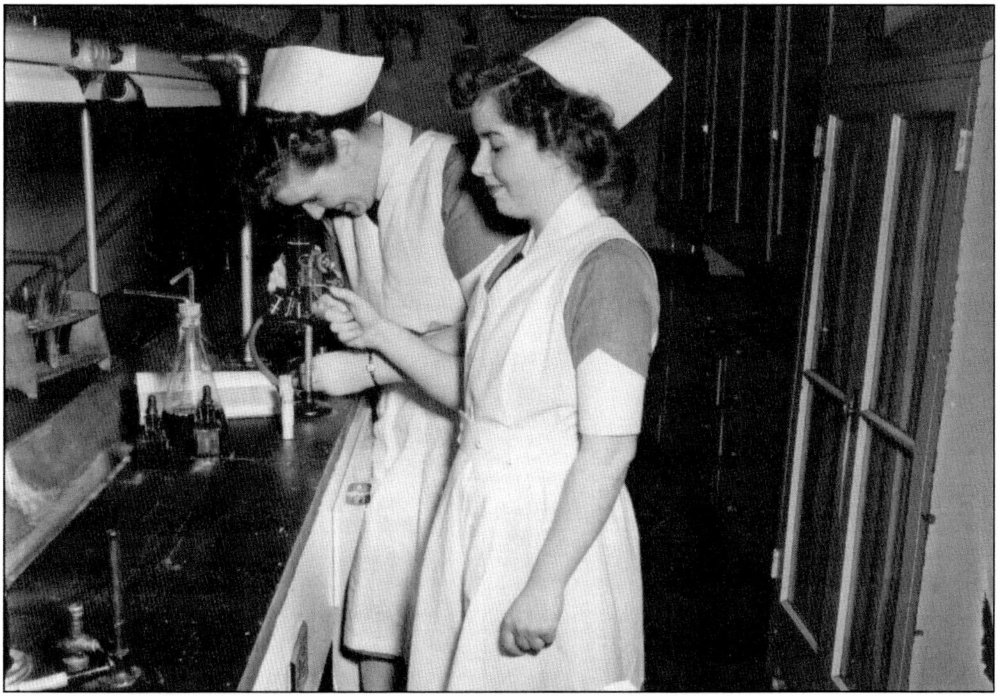

This photograph from 1947 depicts nursing students in the chemistry laboratory in the basement of the Nurses' Residence. A Henry Heywood Memorial School of Nursing alumna says, "I remember one of my classmates lighting the gas jet and forgetting to put the Bunsen burner on first," nearly burning down the building.

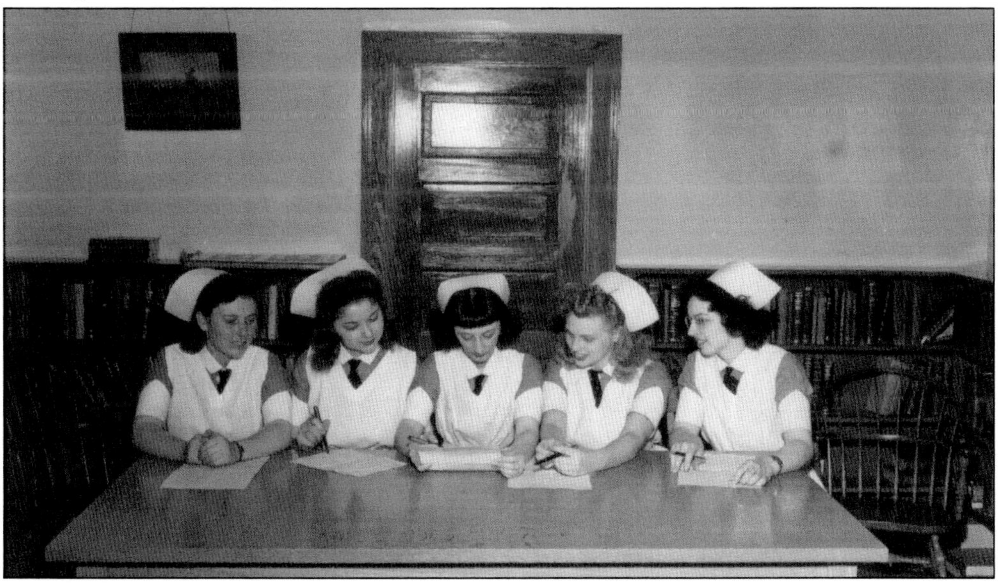

According to a letter from superintendent of nurses M. Adelaide Gilliss, psychometric tests were given to nursing school applicants prior to entrance to eliminate those "unfitted for nursing." Additionally, there was a probationary period for every student. These students from the class of 1949 are studying for a conference. Second from the left is Rosemary Flood, and third from left is Pauline George.

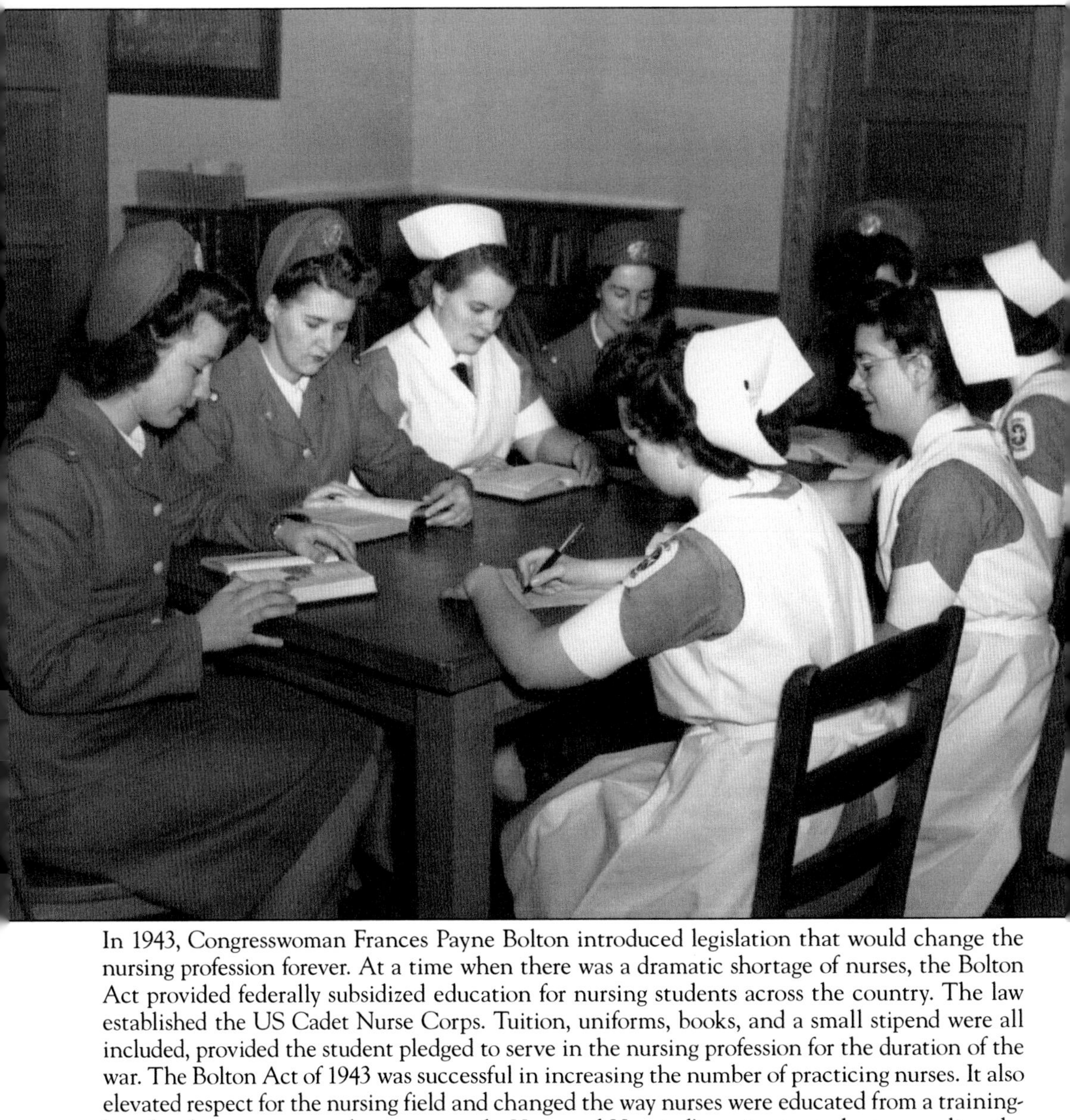

In 1943, Congresswoman Frances Payne Bolton introduced legislation that would change the nursing profession forever. At a time when there was a dramatic shortage of nurses, the Bolton Act provided federally subsidized education for nursing students across the country. The law established the US Cadet Nurse Corps. Tuition, uniforms, books, and a small stipend were all included, provided the student pledged to serve in the nursing profession for the duration of the war. The Bolton Act of 1943 was successful in increasing the number of practicing nurses. It also elevated respect for the nursing field and changed the way nurses were educated from a training-based style to a more academic approach. Heywood Hospital's notice to students regarding the Bolton Act included the stipulation that "a Cadet Corps nurse may plan to marry after graduation if she continues to nurse." In 1944, there were 34 reported alumnae in the US Armed Forces.

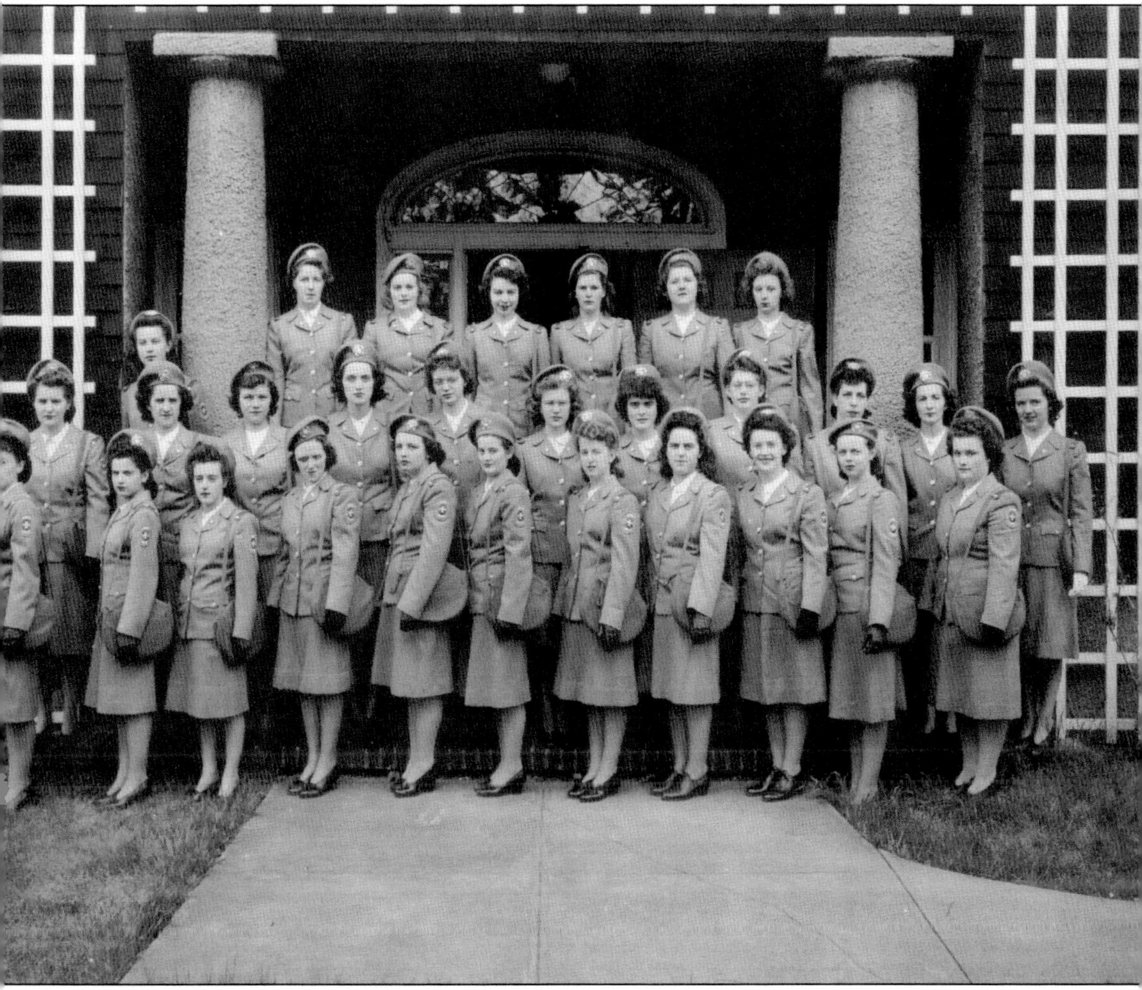

Cadet nurses wore distinctive outdoor uniforms of gray and scarlet. A report from the school of nursing in March 1945 stated that larger classes were being admitted to meet the demand for more nurses. An addition was made to the Nurses' Residence with further residential rooms and a more adequate teaching unit. Interestingly, slightly more than a year later, Henry Heywood Memorial Hospital's director of nursing services wrote to the American Hospital Bureau (AHB) with a plea for assistance in filling nursing positions because of the nationwide shortage. The AHB responded that although they had expected an increasing list of qualified nurses returning from war, "they seem to have no desire to take up the work for which they had been prepared before going into the Army or Navy Nurse Corps and one wonders when they are likely to return to solid earth again." The letter goes on to state, "We just fold our hands and wait . . . until the glamour of having been a Captain or a Major has worn off." The last cadet class registered in September 1945.

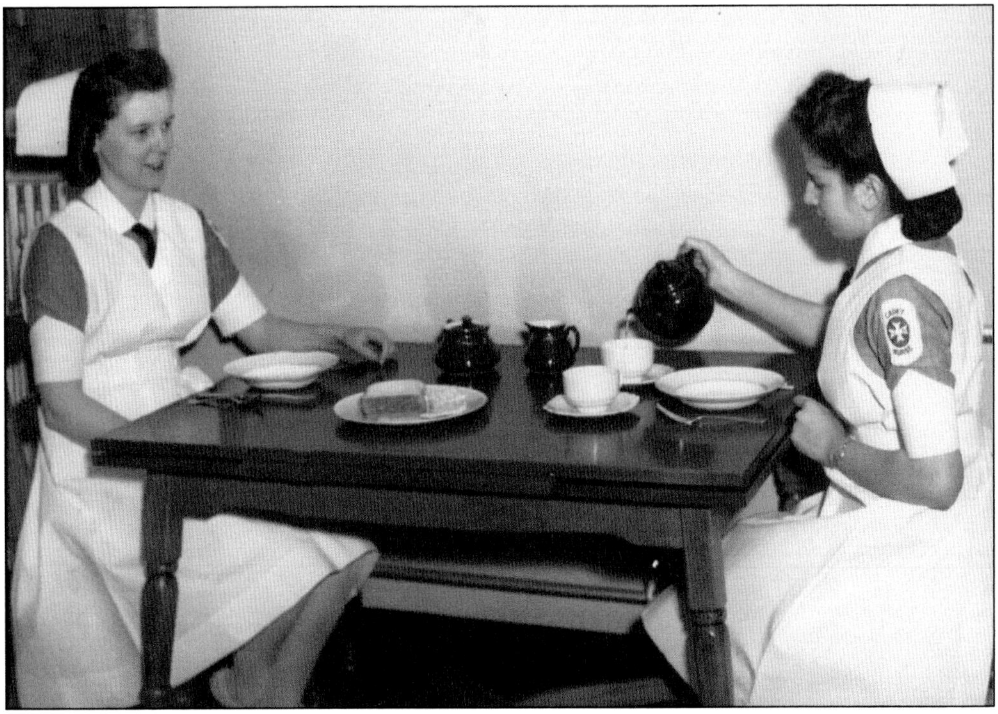

Cadet students Lorraine Knox (left) and Virginia Troy, class of 1947, take a tea break in the kitchen in the basement level of the Nurses' Residence. Knox joined the US Army and was assigned as special nurse to Pres. Dwight Eisenhower while he recovered from a coronary attack at Walter Reed Hospital. The president personally invited Knox to attend the inaugural ball at the White House in 1957.

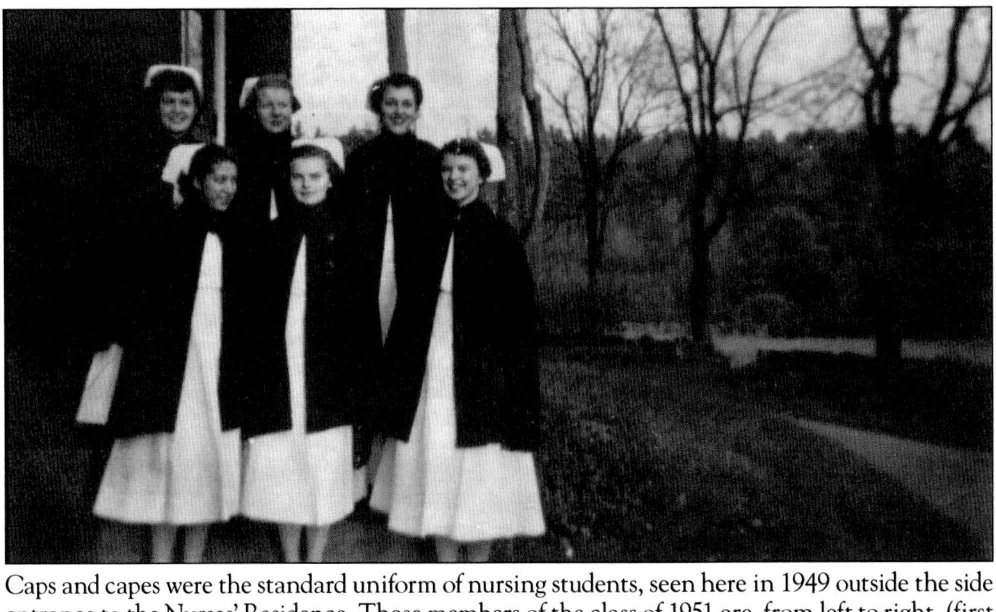

Caps and capes were the standard uniform of nursing students, seen here in 1949 outside the side entrance to the Nurses' Residence. These members of the class of 1951 are, from left to right, (first row) Evelyn Wieres Manyon, Veronica Chojnowski Martel, and Eunice Heald Arcangeli; (second row) Louise Robicaud Frei, Elsie Laurila Baer, and Louise Cormier Nelson.

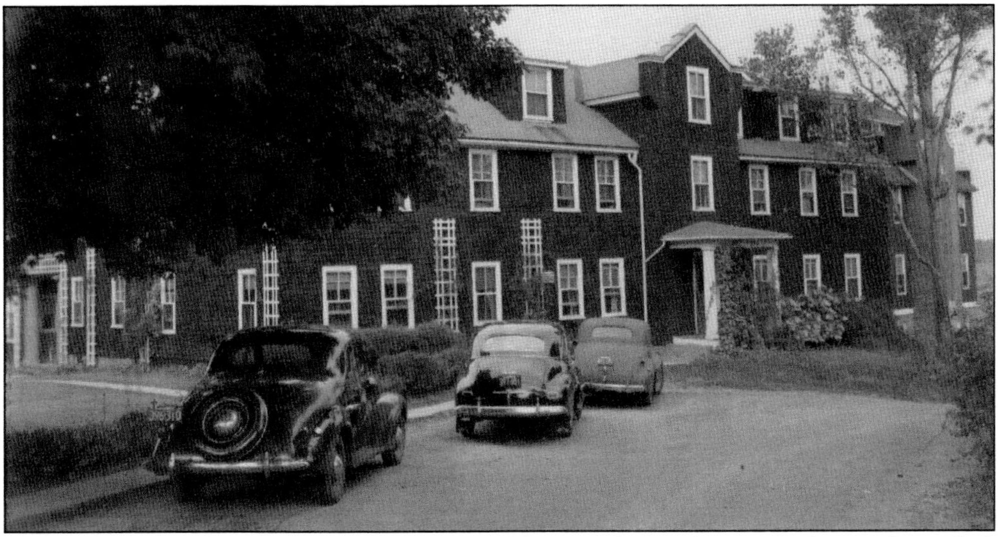

To meet the demand for more nurses during World War II, larger classes were being admitted. A new addition to the Nurses' Residence provided additional sleeping rooms and teaching space. This picture of the now *L*-shaped building was taken in 1946. The housemother's desk was located just inside the main entrance to the left. Students were required to sign in and out upon entering or leaving.

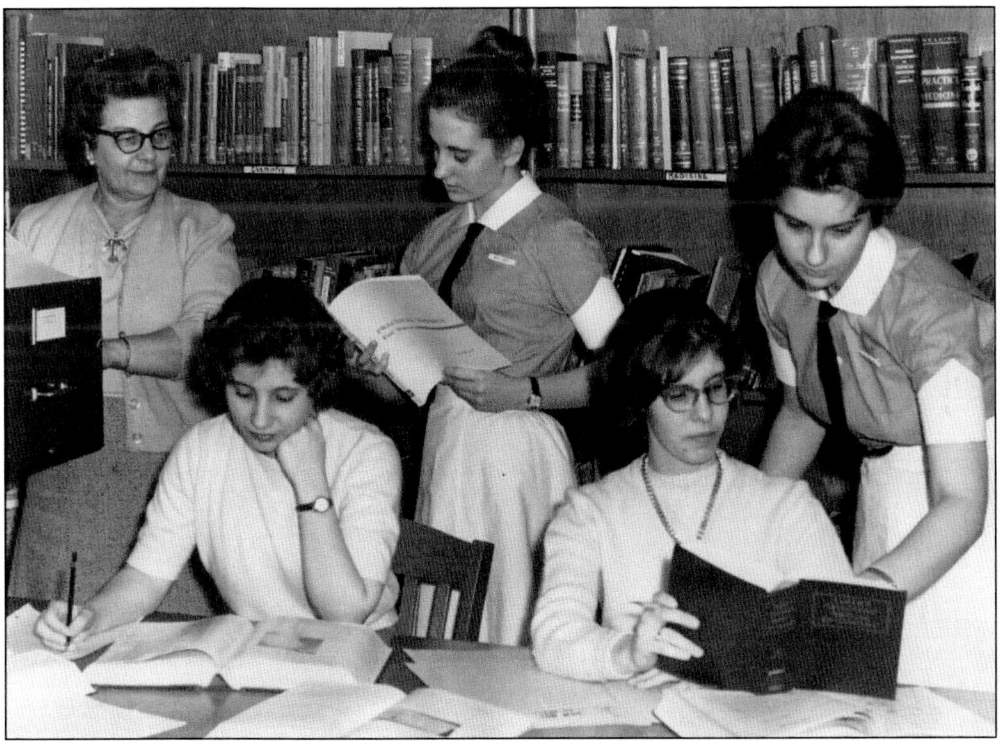

A well-stocked library was provided for the students in the Nurses' Residence. Students were free from 4:00 p.m. until 7:00 p.m. daily but were expected to study from 7:00 p.m. to 9:00 p.m. each evening. This photograph shows a group of students being assisted by librarian Helene Valley in the fall of 1963.

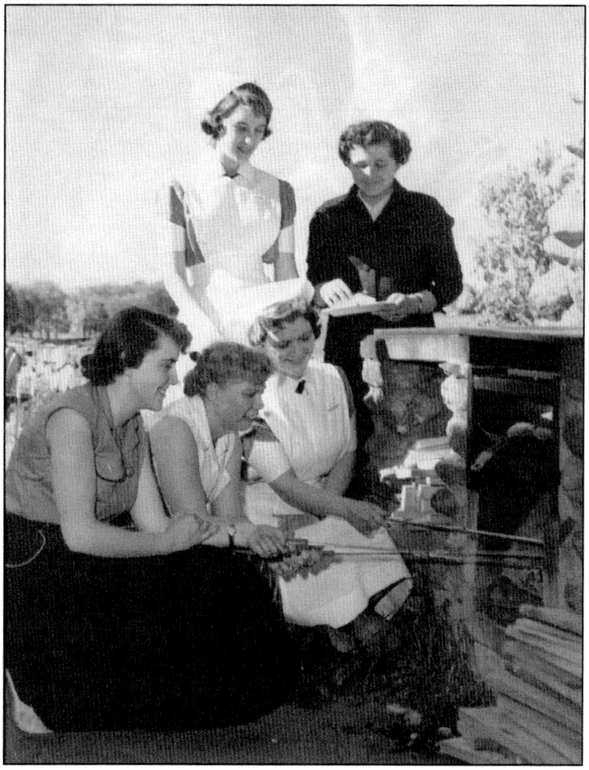

The Nurses' Residence provided room and board for the students as well as a space to study and attend classes. But it was not only a place to live and learn—recreation was plentiful. Cookouts, sports, and dances were among the many activities available to students. It is evident when perusing the reports of the nursing school that student morale was recognized as an important factor. A report from 1945 records activities for the year, such as teas, theater parties, Halloween and Christmas parties, and dances. It also recommends a tennis court be provided for students. Students loved cooking on their new outdoor fireplace behind the residence. Archery was another activity enjoyed by many students. Today, Mount Wachusett Community College and giant wind turbines occupy the field beyond where the students are seen practicing their archery skills.

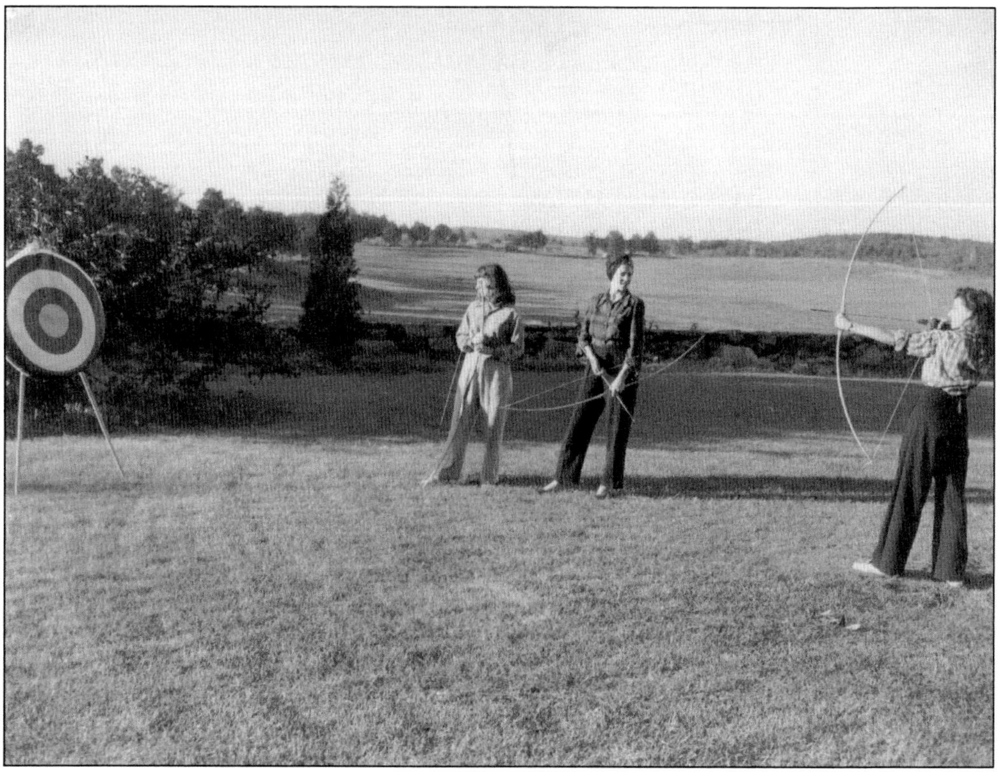

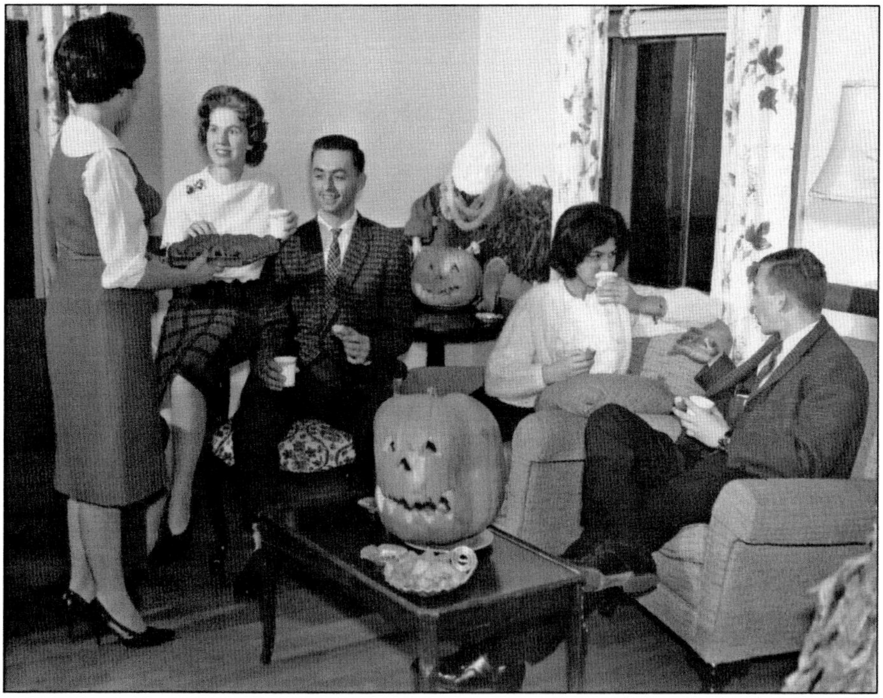

Teas and dances were held in the large common room in the Nurses' Residence. These couples are enjoying cider and donuts at a Halloween dance in the fall of 1962. Barbara Babineau and James Carpenter, the man and woman seated to the left, are now married and live locally. An alumna recalls that with the exception of moving day, boys were *never* allowed past the first floor. Below, nursing students take a recreational trip, most likely to the nearby ski resort at Wachusett Mountain in 1962. Nursing school yearbooks are full of delightful vignettes of how the students lived, worked, and played together during their three years in the program. Identified here looking quite fashionable in their athletic gear are, from left to right, Mary Parnarouskis, Sylvia Adams, Diane Adams, Lynn Tait, and Judith Nielsen.

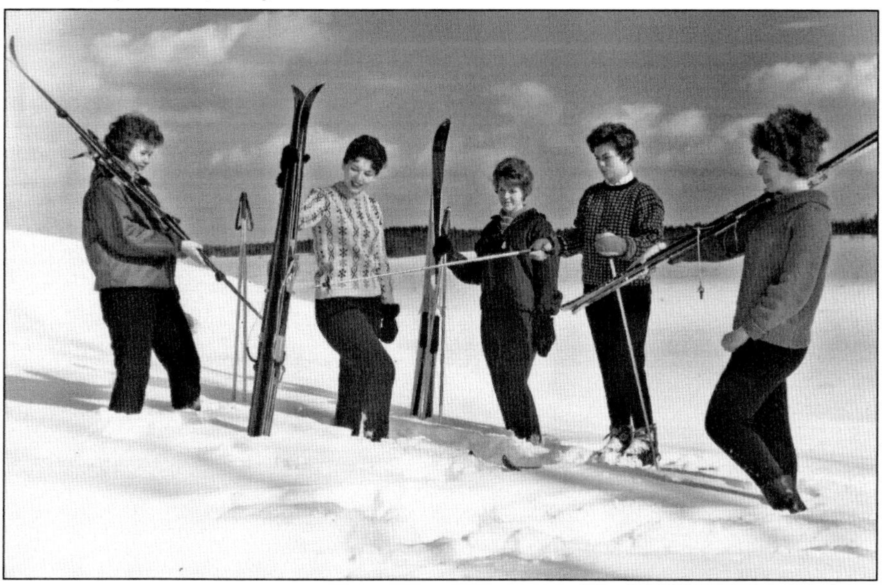

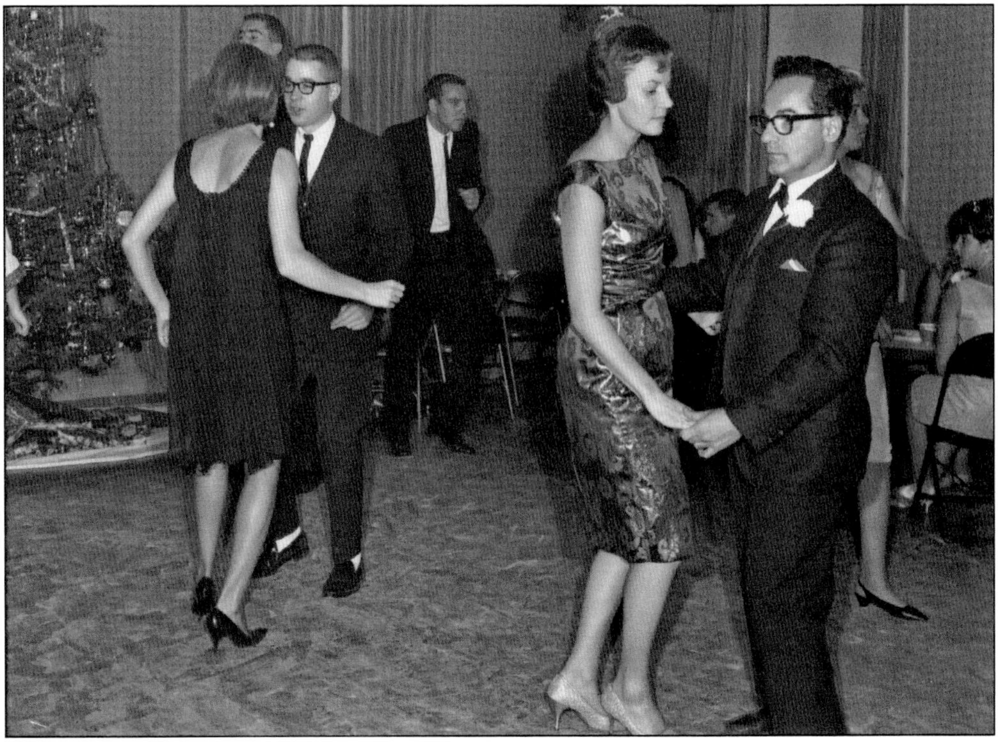

An annual Christmas party was held at the Nurses' Residence. By all accounts, these festivities were enjoyed by all. As chronicled in many nursing school reports, in addition to food and dancing, entertainment might include singing Christmas carols or even a short play. Seen above is a Christmas dance around 1960. The gentleman in the center background is clearly enjoying the dance. Below is a New Year's Eve dance in 1947. Several subjects appear to be camera shy. Obviously a grand occasion, the young women are dressed in their finest gowns, corsages and all.

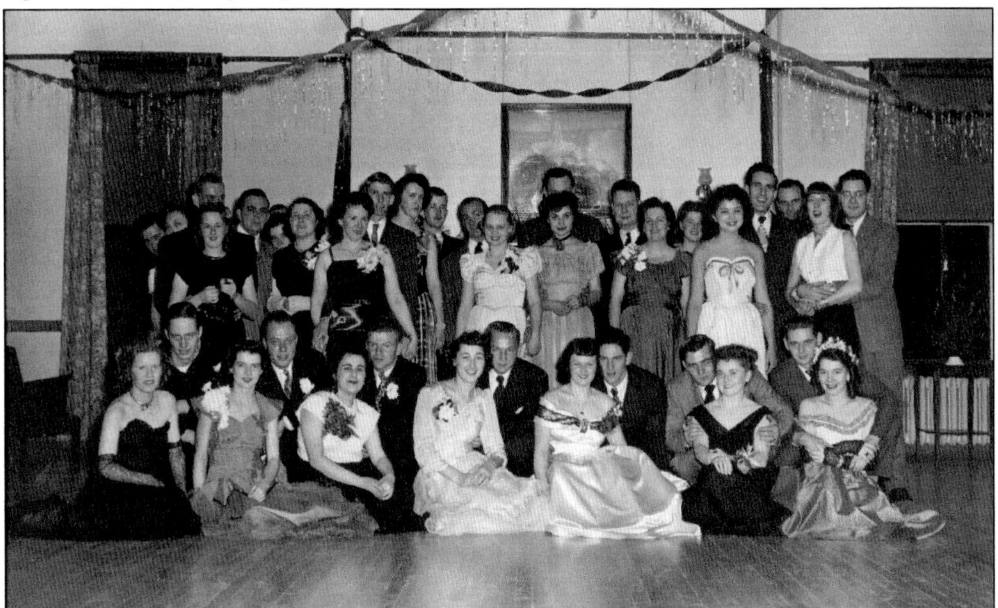

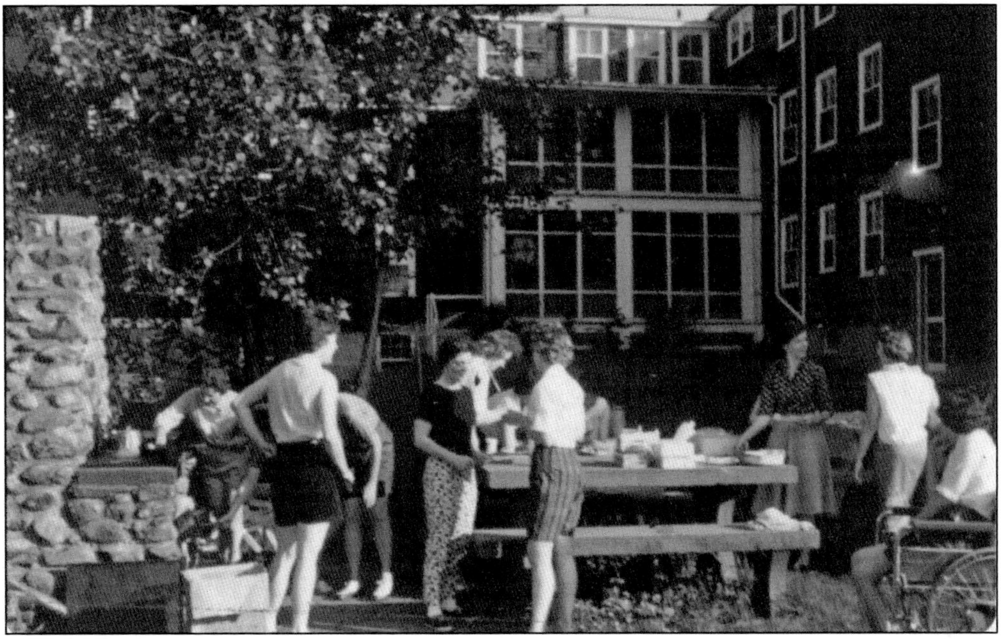

In addition to their clinical training at Henry Heywood Memorial Hospital, nursing students were sent to other area hospitals on affiliation for pediatrics, psychiatric nursing, and communicable disease. Among others, these hospitals included Boston Floating Hospital, Boston City Hospital, Danvers State Hospital, and Providence City Hospital. A communicable disease affiliation became an elective in 1946. Students were routinely vaccinated before being sent for affiliation. Despite this, some students did contract communicable diseases. In the wheelchair on the far right in the above photograph is Marjorie O'Brien, who contracted polio while on affiliation at Boston Floating Hospital. Below, students from the class of 1948 are enjoying an outdoor meal. Upon graduation, Annie Kruglwicz, seen here in the nurse's cap, and two other graduates sought adventure in the wilds of Alaska.

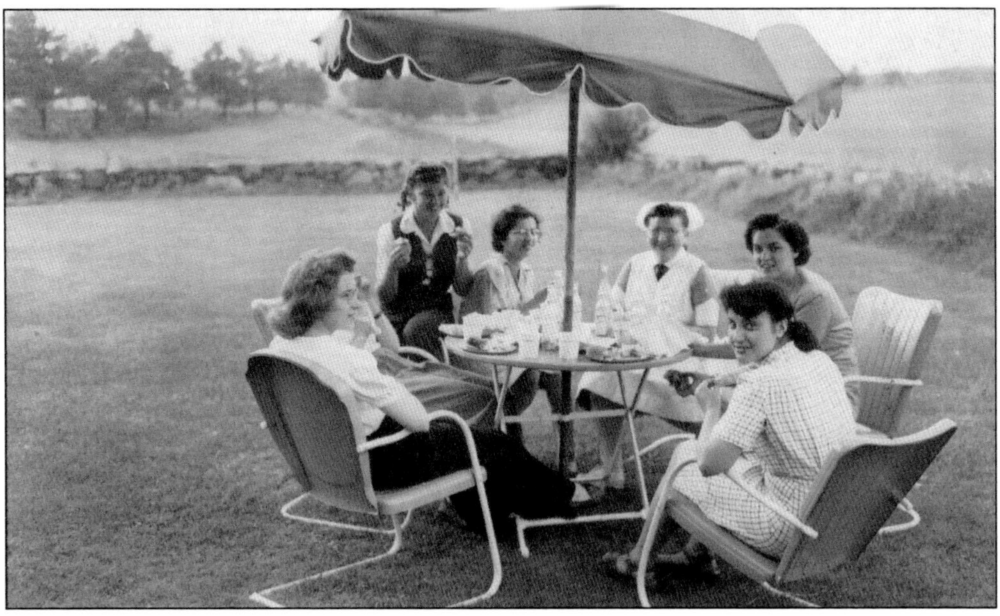

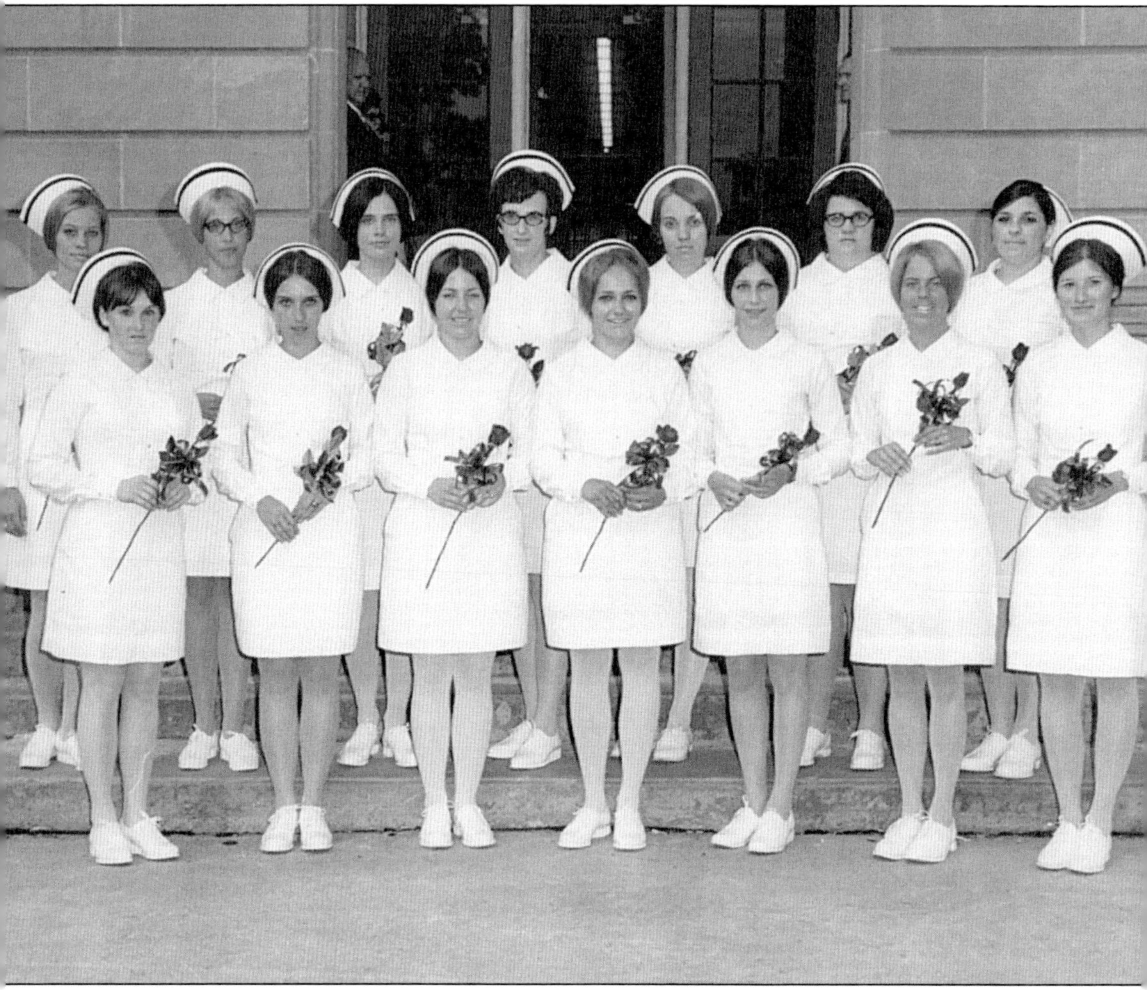

Eventually, the American Nurses Association decreed that the education of licensed nurses must take place in an "institution of higher learning" as opposed to a clinical setting. The last class of nursing students at the Henry Heywood Memorial School of Nursing graduated in 1970. Hospital administrator Harold Callahan lamented the closure. According to the Heywood Hospital Nursing Alumnae Association, a total of 638 students graduated from the program over the 41 years it was in existence. Featured here in the last class photograph ever taken are, alphabetically by maiden name, Sheila Botti Powiliatis, Andrea Boucher Goulding Mitchell, Teresa Golec, Gail Grimes, Louise LaFlamme Hashway, Roberta Mailloux Lajoie, Suzanne McComish Rogstad, Laurie Millar King, Carolyn Murdock Malecko, Nancy Oberg, Patricia O'Brien, Catherine Phillips Fontaine, Patricia Storti Croteau, and Donna Zera. Today, Heywood Hospital hosts nursing students fulfilling their clinical coursework from nearby institutions such as Mount Wachusett Community College and Fitchburg State College.

Five

Rapid Fire Renovations in 1961–1971

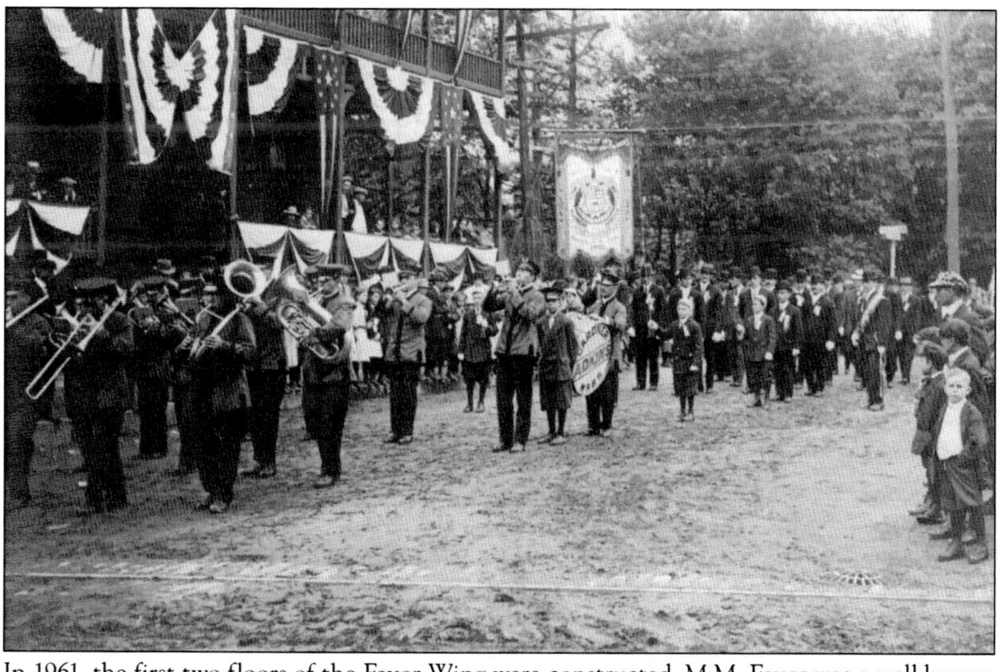

In 1961, the first two floors of the Favor Wing were constructed. M.M. Favor was a well-known builder in Gardner. He owned and operated the Favor Lumber Company. A marching band is shown in front of the Commercial House. Located at the corner of Parker Street and West Street, the Commercial House was built by Favor in 1897. (Courtesy of GM.)

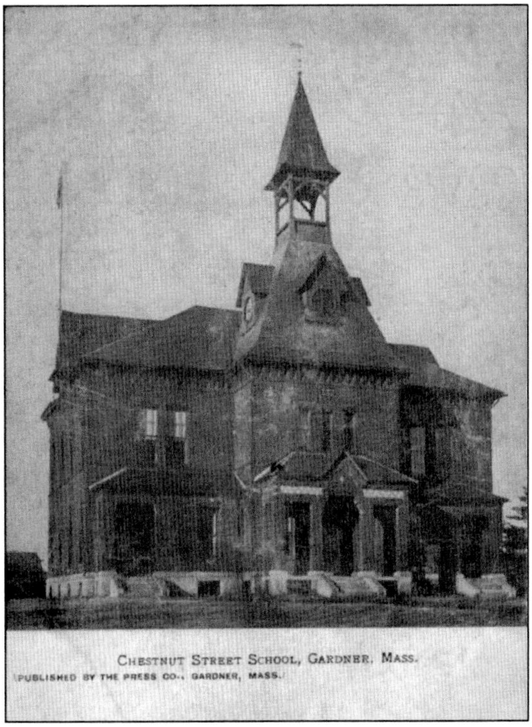

M.M. Favor was a unique builder in that he had the skills to design the structure, supply the materials, and construct the building. Favor constructed prominent buildings, such as the furniture factories for S. Bent and Brothers and Nichols and Stone. This image is of the Chestnut Street High School built by Favor in 1874. (Courtesy of GM.)

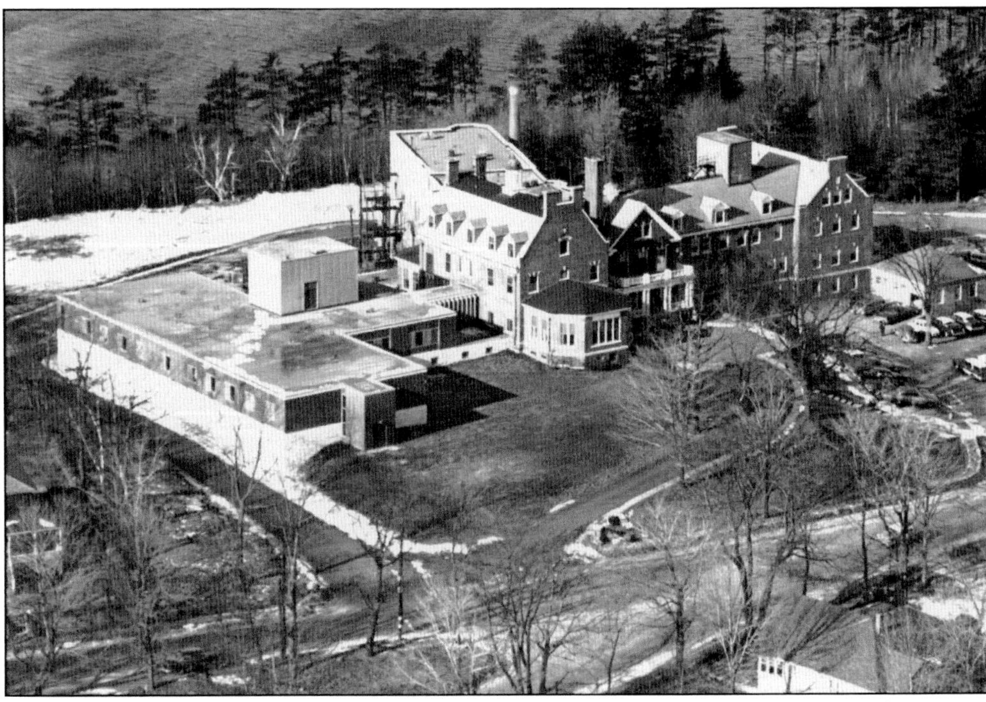

Frank M. Favor was the philanthropist son of M.M. Favor. He willed an amount of money to Heywood Hospital that was second only to Martha Heywood's donation. The Favor Fund was earmarked to cover the medical bills of patients who could not afford the payments. The Favor Wing was built in two sections—the first two floors in 1961 and the next two stories in 1971.

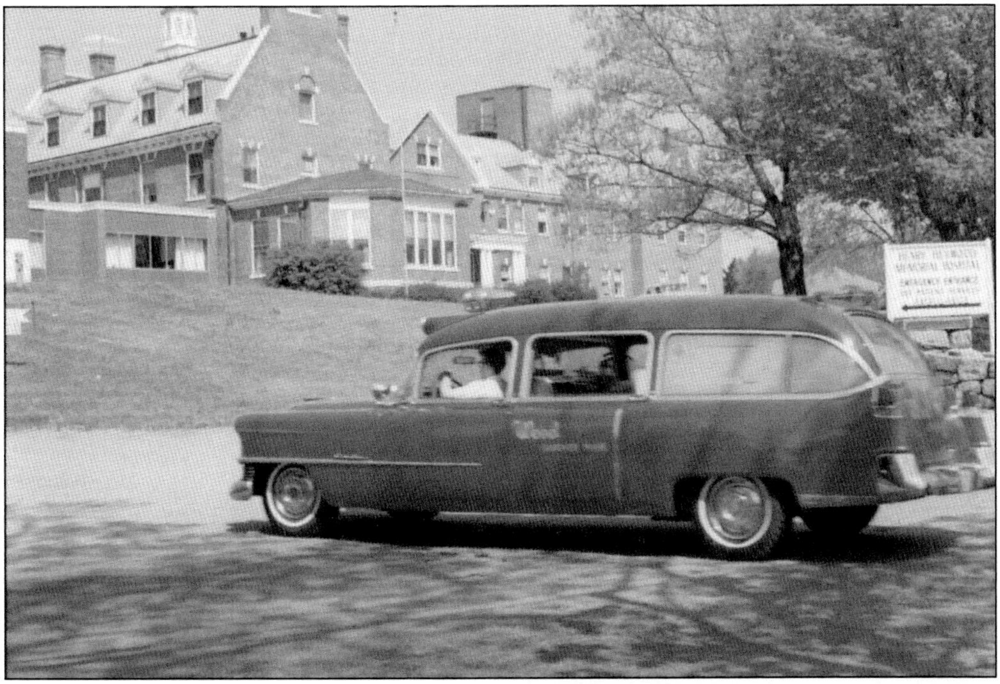

The ground floor of the Favor Wing contained an emergency room and surgical suite. The emergency room had four rooms separated by accordion dividers. The ambulance entrance shared the patient entrance. The ambulance patients on stretchers had to be wheeled past the waiting room. The surgical suite had six operating rooms. Operating rooms one and two were the main rooms used for major cases, such as bowel resections. The third room was for eye cases, the fourth for dental cases and tonsillectomies, the fifth for cystoscopies, and the sixth for outpatient surgeries—the forerunner of "surgical day" cases. At right, Dr. Joseph Forte (center) is performing surgery. (Right, courtesy of Dr. Joseph Forte.)

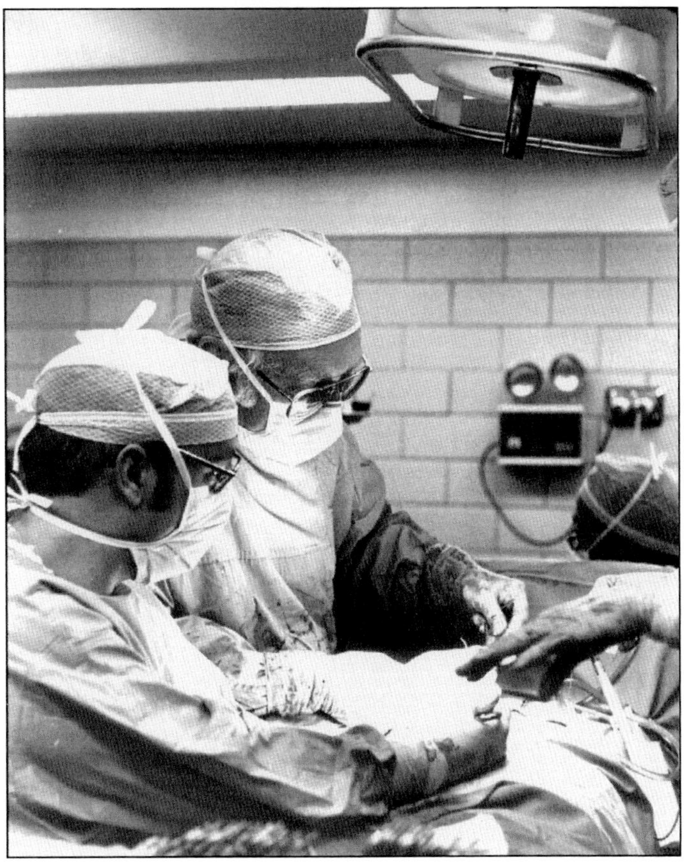

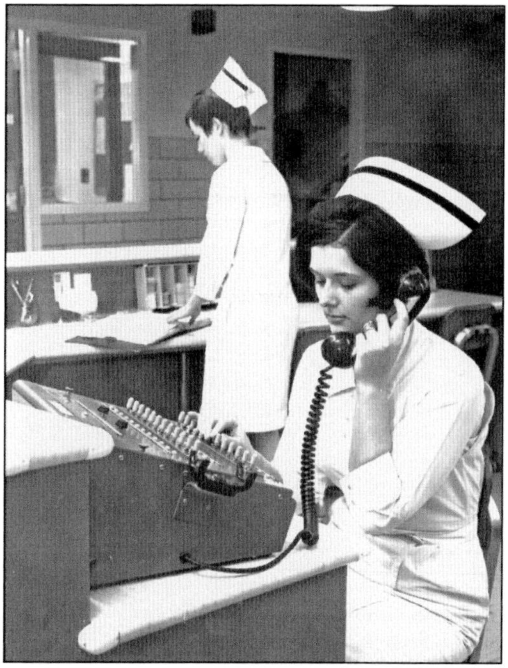

The first floor was called Favor I. A large central nursing station was surrounded by two four-bed wards, semiprivate rooms, and a few single rooms. This floor took the place of the medical-surgical floor on the second floor of the North Wing. This image shows the new central nursing station.

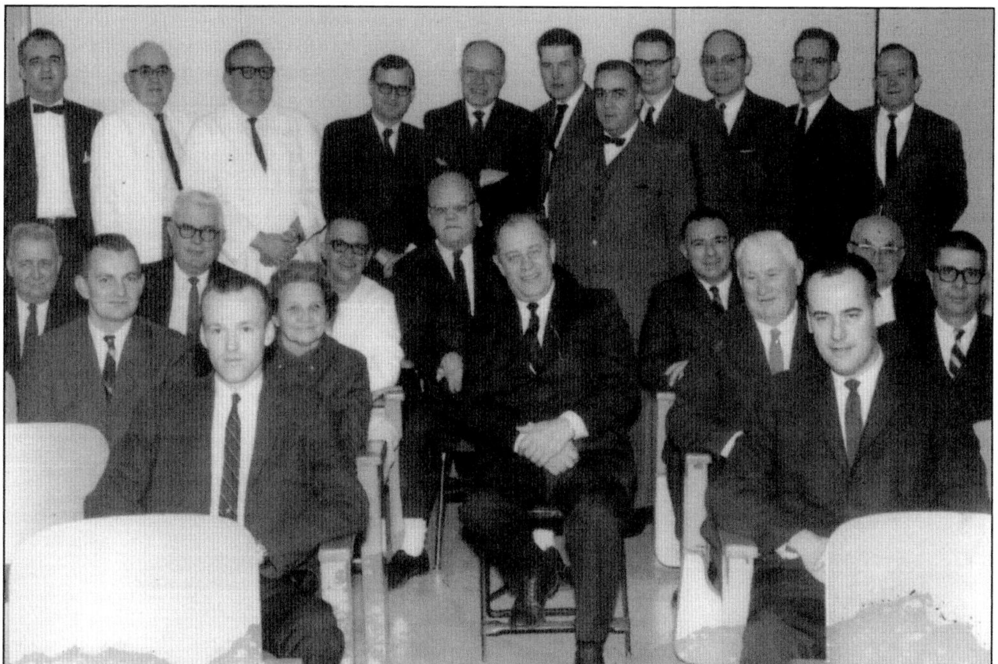

Physicians practicing here in the 1960s include, from left to right, (seated) T. Roland Ekwall, Don Miller, Joe Marnane, Elmer Dech, Beatrice Perkins, Bill Wilson, Paul Dunn, Al Blouin, Rocco Raduazo, Paul Harasimowicz, Bill Damon, Leonard Thompson, and Aubrey Gould; (standing) Terrance Hogan, Clarence McPeak, Mike Smalkin, Max Frei, Dieter Keller, Tom Tracy, Trento Domenici, Jim Faust, Joe Forte, John Mason, and Owen Christensen. (Courtesy of Dr. Joseph Forte.)

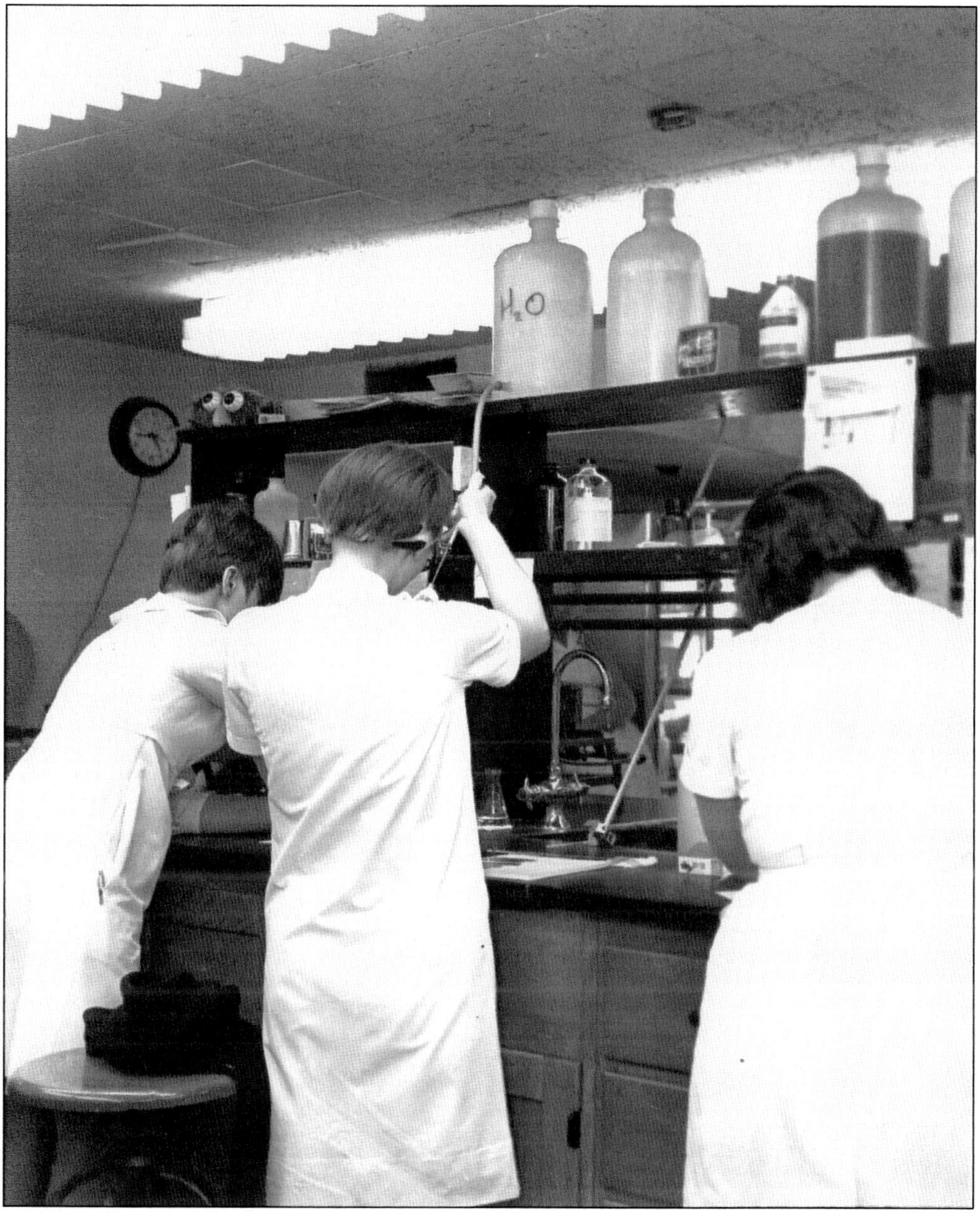

During the 1960s, the laboratory occupied a few rooms in the connector between the original 1907 building and the West Wing. All urine testing was performed by one person—Impi Sylvester—and no one else. There were no phlebotomists. All laboratory technicians drew the blood as well as performed the testing. The average daily volume was 25 complete blood counts (CBC), 35 chemistry tests, 10 coagulation tests, 20 urinalyses, and 25 cultures for a total of 115 tests per day. This was considered "brutally busy." Pipetting was done by mouth. Chemicals added to urine were pipetted. Gloves were not worn. Blood donors were not paid in cash, but were offered a shot of whiskey if desired. When human immunosuppressive virus (HIV) was discovered in the mid-1980s, safety precautions improved. Automation and analyzers increased productivity. In 2007, over one million procedures were done. Seen here are laboratory technicians, with one using a pipette.

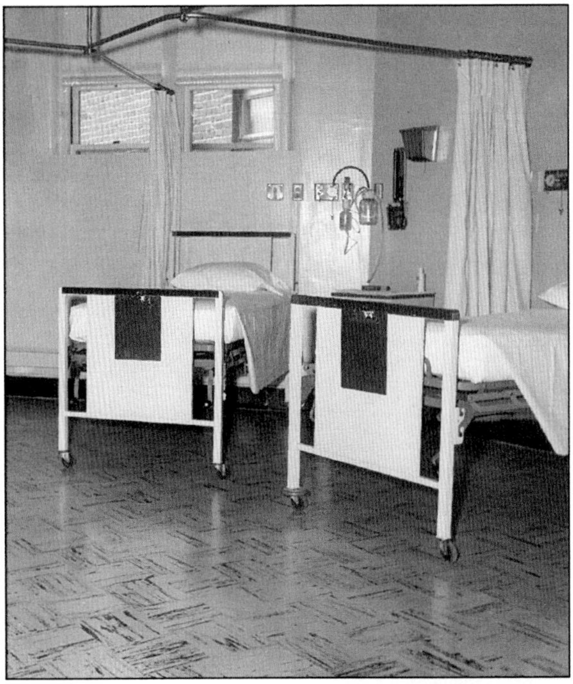

The original intensive care unit (ICU) opened in 1965 under the direction of Dr. Trento Domenici, a board-certified internist. This entailed educating physicians and nurses in cardio-pulmonary resuscitation and identification and treatment of cardiac arrhythmias. An astute clinician, he set the standards for the physicians and nurses in the ICU. A portrait of Domenici hangs in the ICU in his honor. At that time, the ICU occupied the original female ward and consisted of one private room and a five-bed ward. The image at left shows two of the ICU beds. The original 1907 ward is recognizable by the octagonal shape of the room. The oxygen and suction units on the wall and the beds are new to the section. The photograph below is of Dr. Trento Domenici and his wife Beatrice.

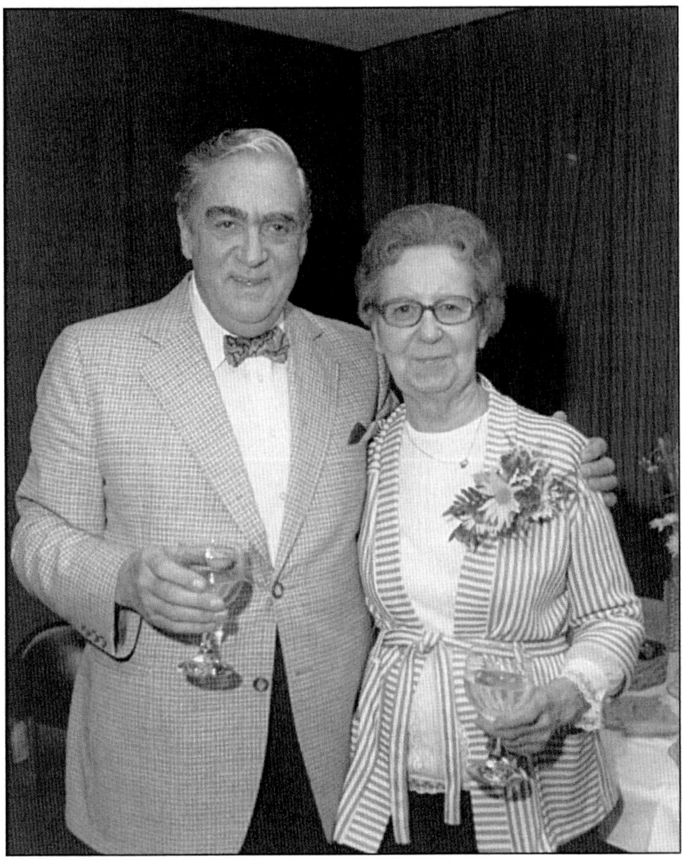

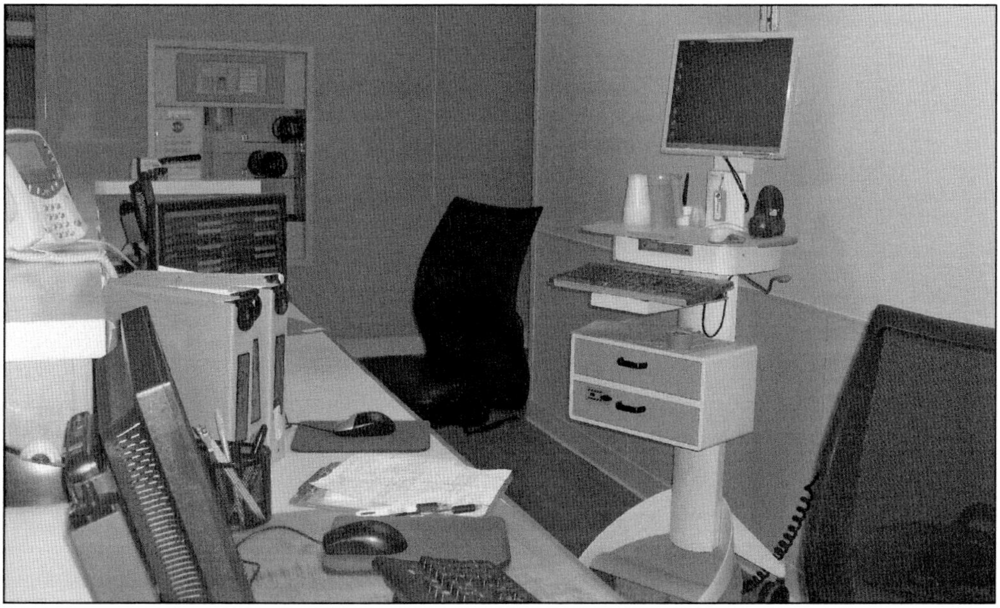

Ten years after the Favor Wing was built, two more floors were added. Named Favor II and Favor III, the wings were essentially the same. Favor III contained a new telemetry unit and ICU. This provided more patient rooms. In addition, the telemetry and ICU units brought Heywood Hospital up to date in terms of treating cardiac patients. Shown above is a modern central monitoring system for a telemetry unit, which enabled the nurses to detect abnormal heart rates and rhythms and monitor vital signs. Below is the finished Favor Wing building. The white-brick ground floor housed the emergency room and surgical suite. The top three floors were dedicated to cardiac, medical, and surgical care. Attached to the southern side of the original 1907 structure, it is a formidable tribute to humanitarian Frank Favor.

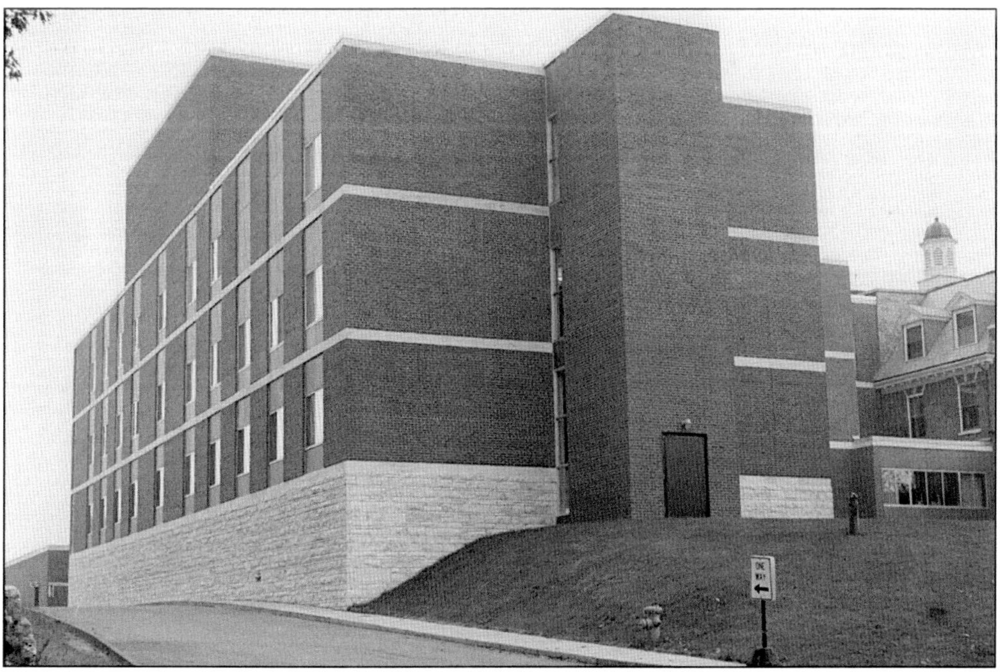

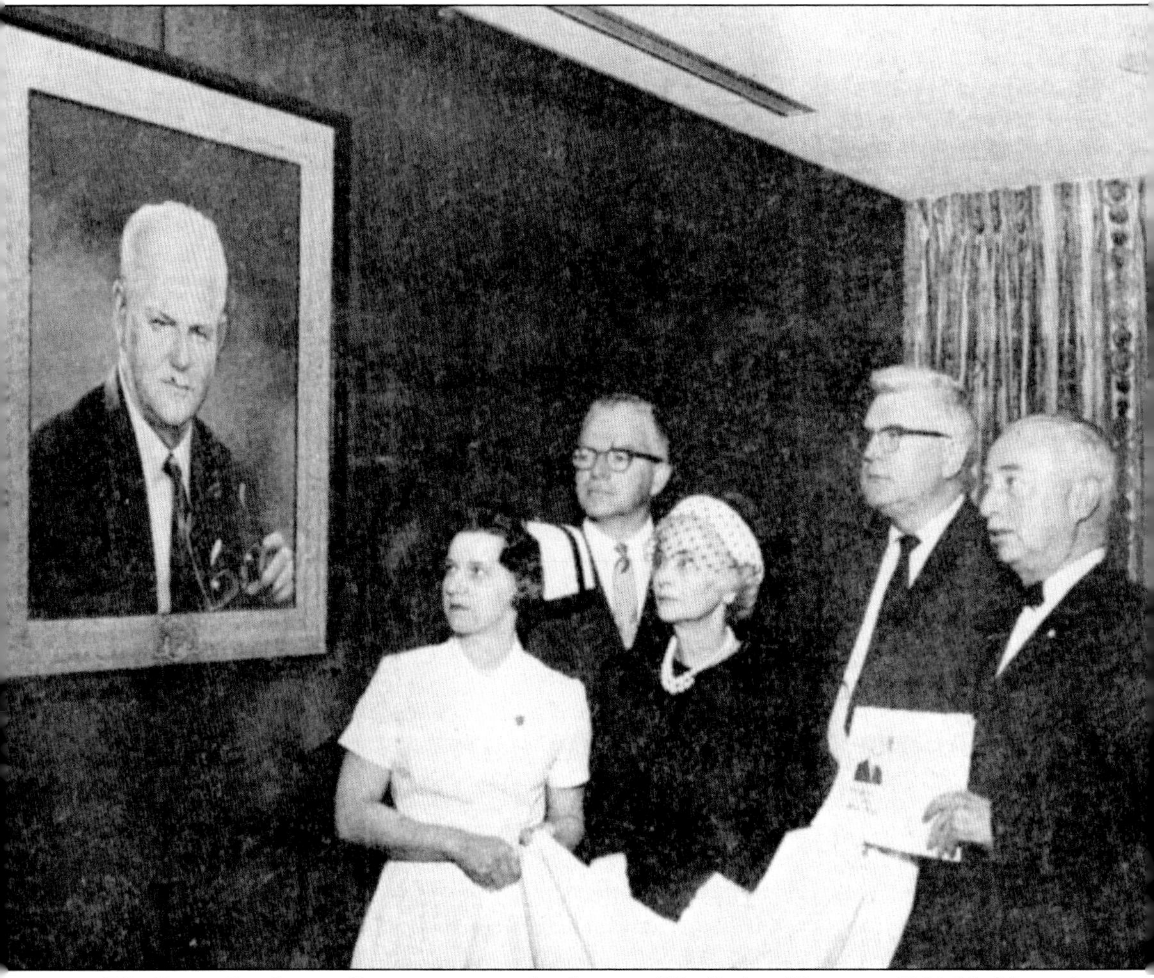

The Pierce Conference Room was erected in honor of Dr. Richard Pierce in 1964. Visible in the bottom photograph on page 63, it was originally located between the Favor Wing and the original 1907 hospital with a bank of windows facing east. A graduate of Harvard College and Harvard Medical School, Pierce joined Heywood Hospital's surgical staff in 1938. During World War II, Pierce was separated from his family for 42 straight months while he served his country as an Army major in the 105th General Hospital unit in the Pacific Islands. His many accomplishments include an article (entitled "Problems with a Small Community Hospital") coauthored with colleague Dr. Trento Domenici in 1963 for the *New England Journal of Medicine*. Present for the unveiling of Pierce's portrait at the dedication of the conference room are, from left to right, head surgical nurse Margaret Roy, Mrs. Richard Pierce, chief of surgery Dr. Joseph Marnane, Curtis Watkins, and chairman of the board Charles Brooks. (Courtesy of the *Gardner News*.)

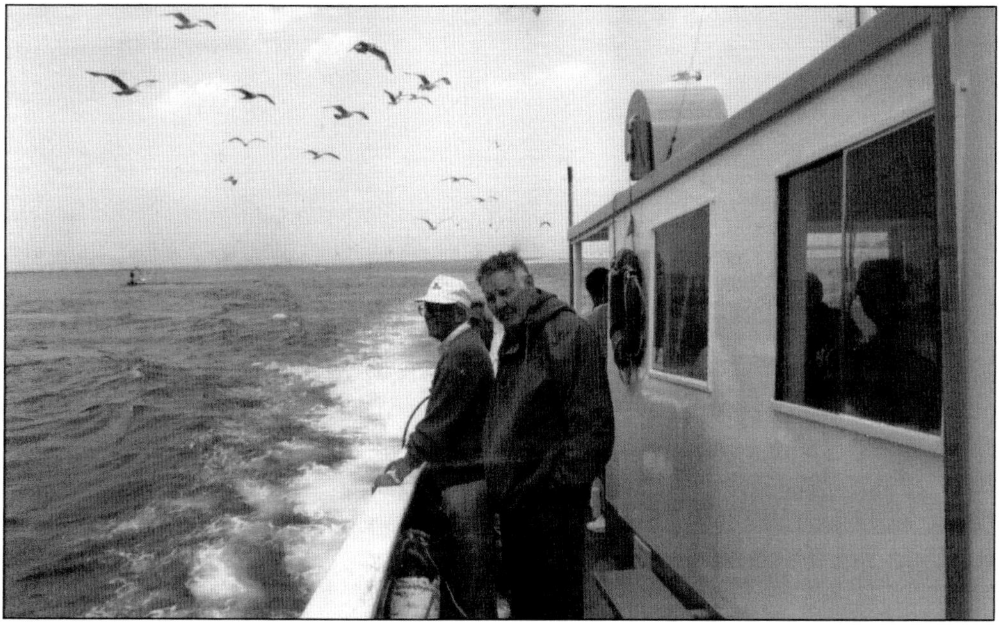

The Pierce Conference Room became the daily meeting place for physicians between morning rounds and office hours. Physician camaraderie, a trademark of the small community hospital, was enhanced. Physicians annually took fishing trips together. Featured here are Dr. Bill Wilson (left) and Dr. Tom Tracy with a group of colleagues on a fishing trip off the coast of Cape Cod. (Courtesy of Dr. John Skrzypczak.)

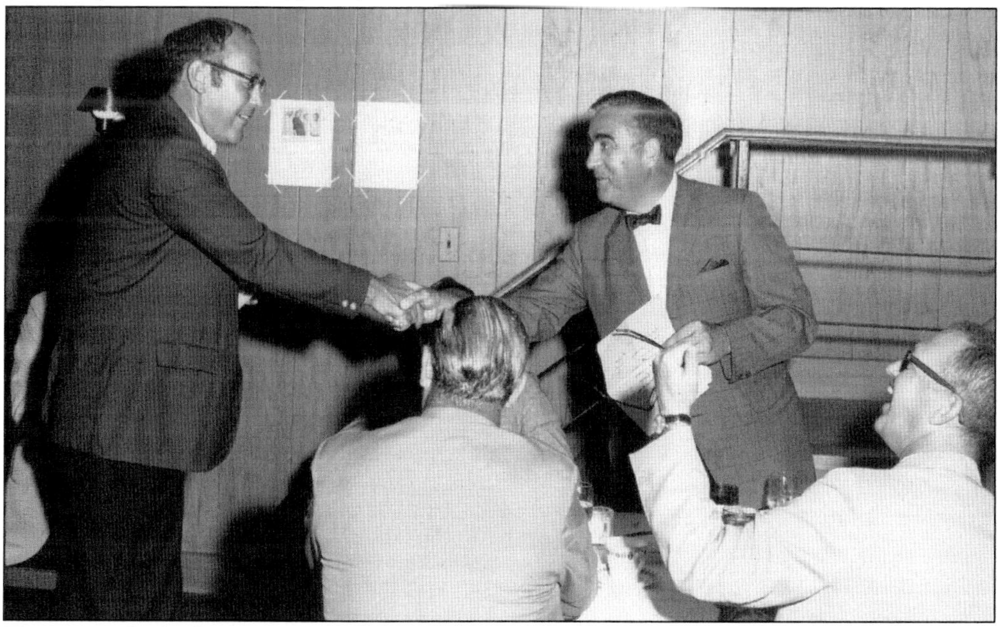

Physicians also had an annual golf tournament with Burbank Hospital at Oak Hill Country Club in nearby Fitchburg, Massachusetts. The two hospitals shared many specialists. In this photograph, Dr. Joseph Forte (left) accepts congratulations from Dr. Trento Domenici for the best net golf score. Looking on are Dr. Al Blouin (center) and Bill Wilson (right). Of note is that Forte had a handicap of 36. (Courtesy of Dr. Joseph Forte.)

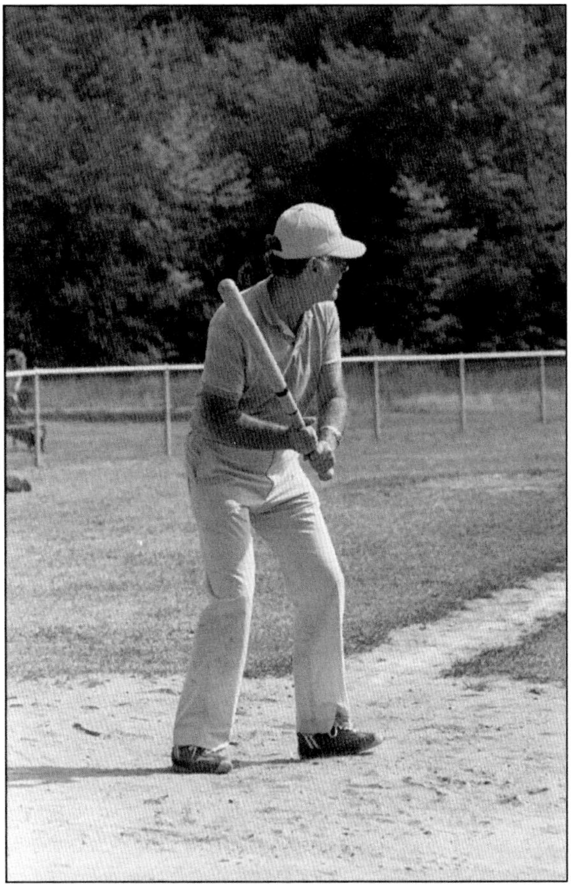

An annual hockey game that pitted physicians against city employees was referred to as the "Saint Valentine's Day Massacre." On Saturday, February 21, 1976, the score was tied three to three when city employee Lou Martin and physician Jack Siarnacki each scored a goal, leaving it a deadlock. However, the good will gained was a winner for all. Heywood Hospital physicians also played an annual Labor Day softball game for charity. Their opponents were the Gardner City Hall employees. The slugger in the image at left is Dr. Joseph Forte. Below is the next generation of sluggers, the Mighty Docs. (Left, courtesy of Dr. Joseph Forte; below, courtesy of Dr. John Skrzypczak.)

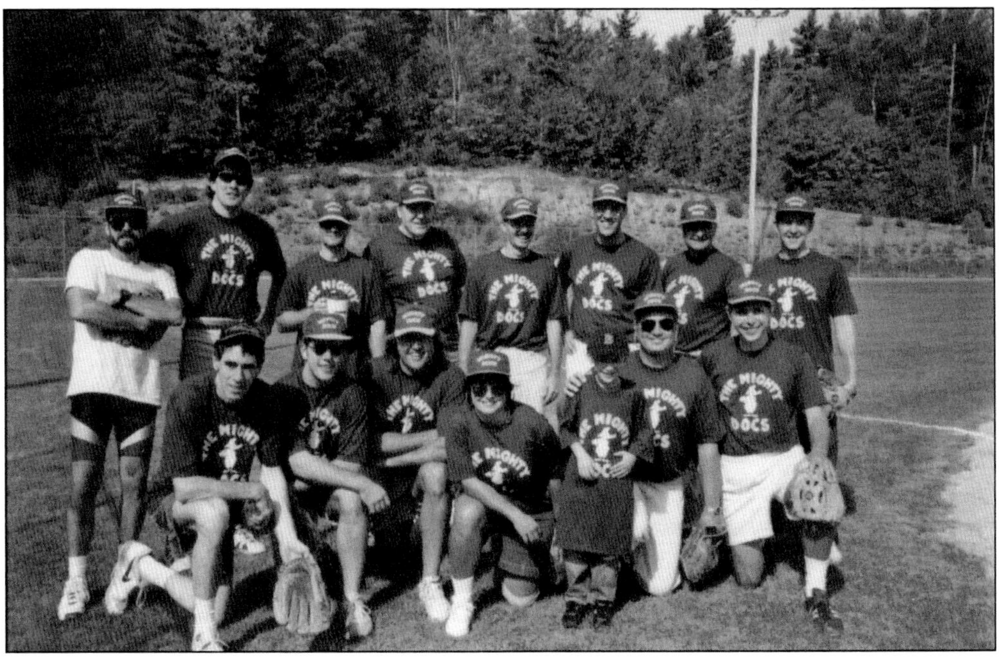

Six

Disaster Drills

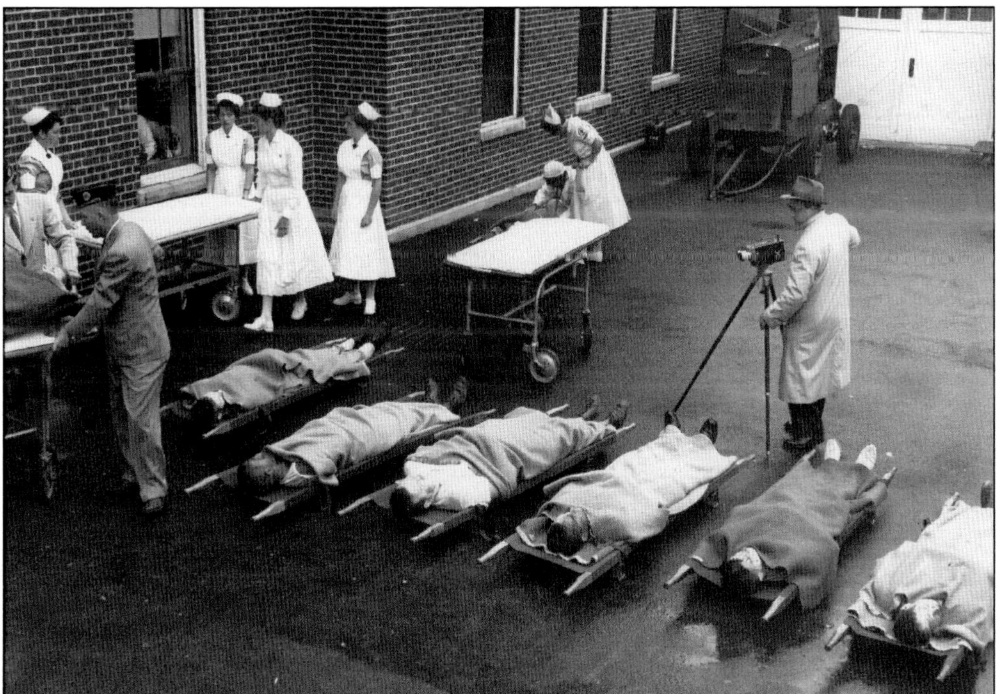

The year 1957 was when Henry Heywood Memorial Hospital celebrated its 50th anniversary. It was also the year the hospital produced the film *Disaster Plan*. Members of the hospital staff wrote the script and oversaw the project. Professionally filmed by the Bay State Film Company, it was the first film of its kind to be produced and was used by other hospitals across the nation to train personnel in disaster preparedness.

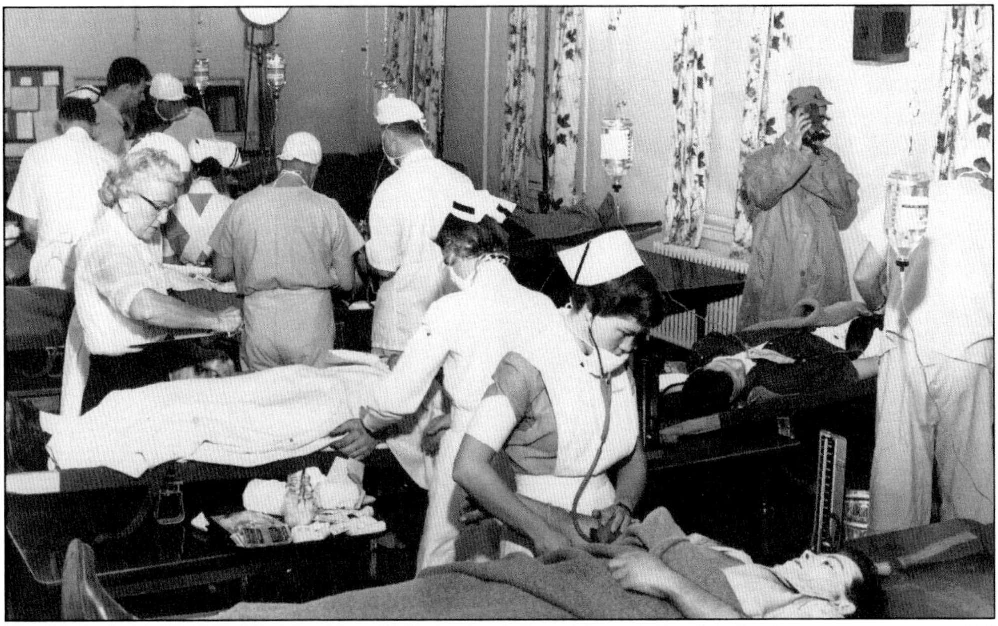

The original script was written and the movie shot. To get the final 15-minute version, 2.5 hours of film was edited. According to the film advisory committee, *Disaster Plan* was reviewed by many experts in the field of disaster planning with not a single adverse comment. They also noted that although audio technology of the era allowed easy deletion of a word, inserting one was nearly impossible.

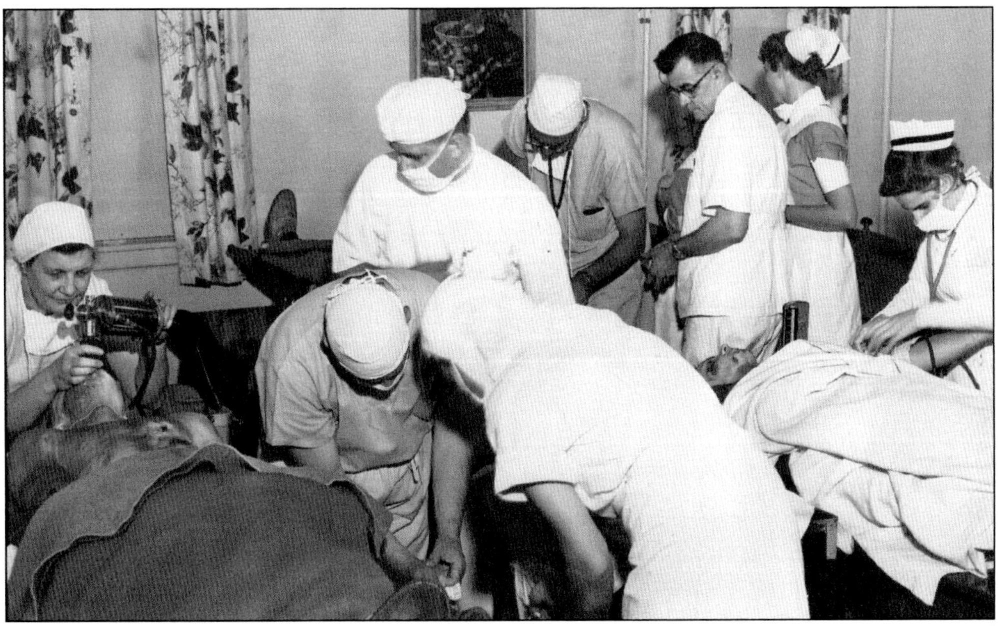

Written in 1957, the hospital's original disaster plan was the joint effort of Henry Heywood Memorial Hospital, the American Red Cross, and the Civil Defense Department. Realizing that the hospital would be unable to provide sufficient personnel and supplies to care for large numbers of casualties in the case of a disaster, these organizations joined forces, drew up the plan, and pledged their commitment to designated responsibilities.

Paul T. Driscoll was the chairman of the disaster committee for the Gardner Chapter of the American Red Cross in 1957. In this image, a poster advertises the Red Cross Bloodmobile coming to the Gardner Elks Club to collect lifesaving blood products to provide to the hospital. Close inspection reveals that one of the books on the table is entitled *When Disaster Strikes*.

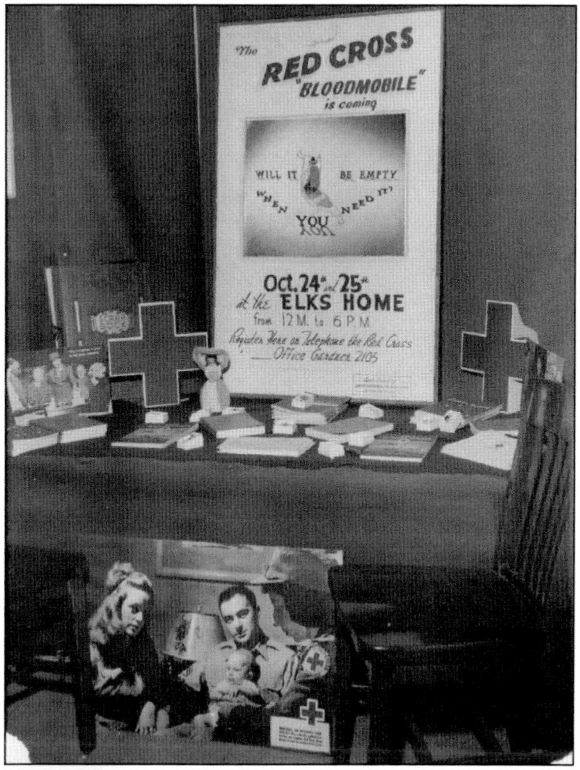
The
RED CROSS
"BLOODMOBILE"
is coming
WILL IT BE EMPTY
WHEN YOU NEED IT?
Oct. 24th and 25th
at the ELKS HOME
from 12 M. to 6 P.M.
Register Here or Telephone the Red Cross
Office Gardner 2105

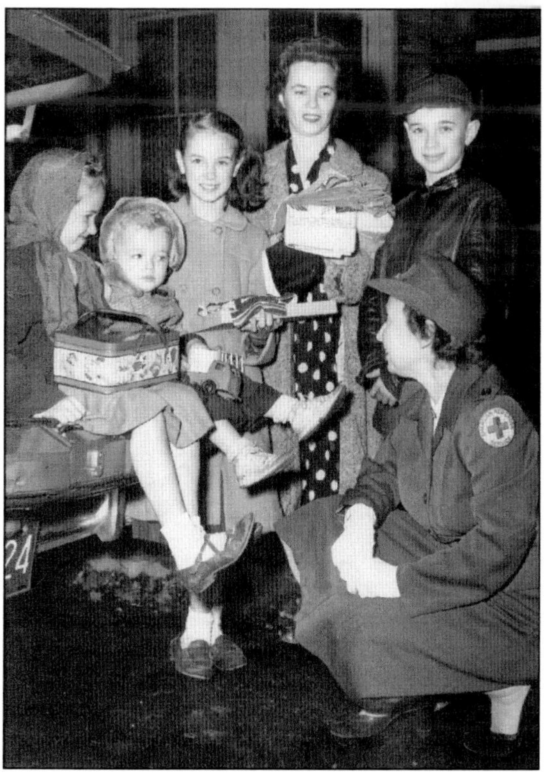

The chief of the Information Center was designated to notify the Red Cross in the case of a disaster. In addition to providing blood products for casualties during an event, the disaster plan designated the Red Cross to handle all incoming calls dealing with inquiries concerning patients and their families. Red Cross "feeding teams" assisted in providing fluids and meals for patients and coffee and doughnuts for personnel.

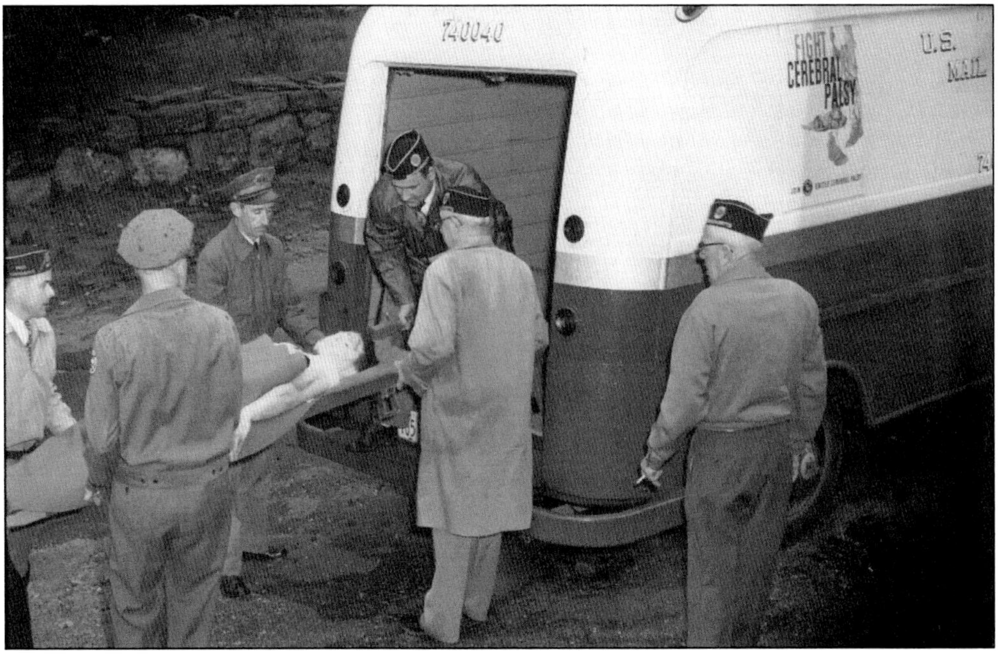

During an event, the hospital must have close communication and partnership with multiple organizations. Here, members of the local American Legion and the US Postal Service are part of the "litter team." A postal delivery truck is doubling as an ambulance. If the need arose, the 1957 disaster plan called for an emergency blood bank to be set up at the local American Legion.

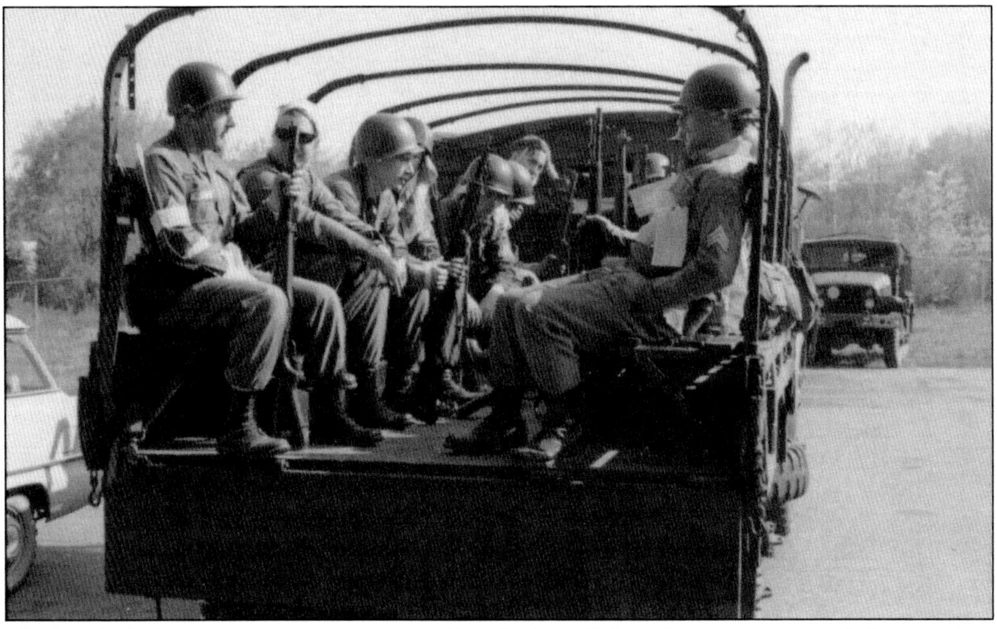

The hospital administrator at that time was Harold A. Callahan. He was responsible for notifying local Civil Defense Department director Philip S. Holmes of a disaster alert. Controlling traffic, transporting casualties, and keeping order were among the responsibilities of these men. In the 1950s and 1960s, the United States was in the midst of the Cold War, and interest in civil defense practices was high.

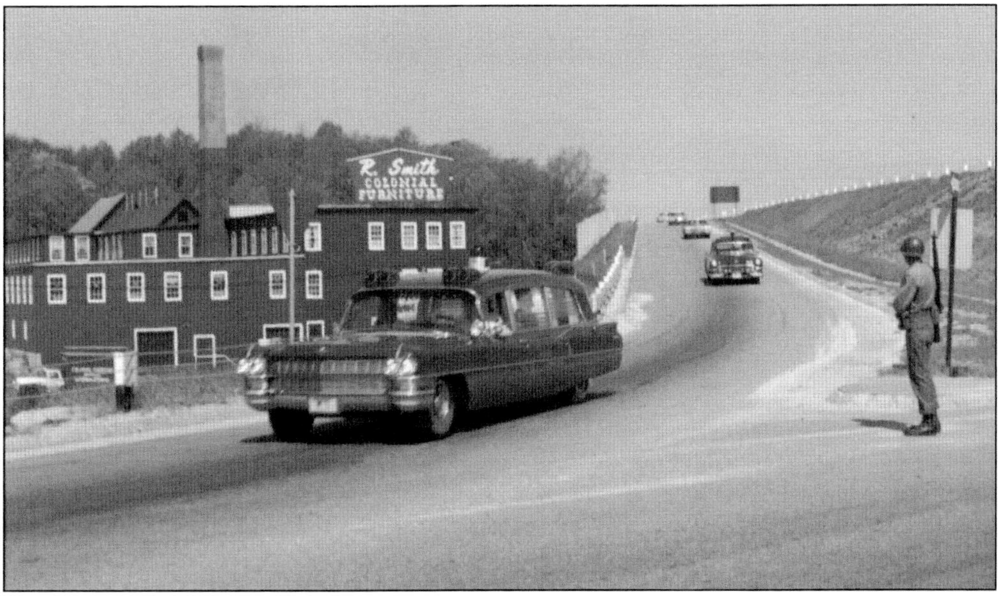

With a disaster drill in progress, a Civil Defense Department member is seen above at his post. These men reported to the hospital administrator but were supervised by the chief of maintenance. The ambulances are exiting Route 2 via Exit 23 and are passing in front of R. Smith Furniture Company, founded in 1956.

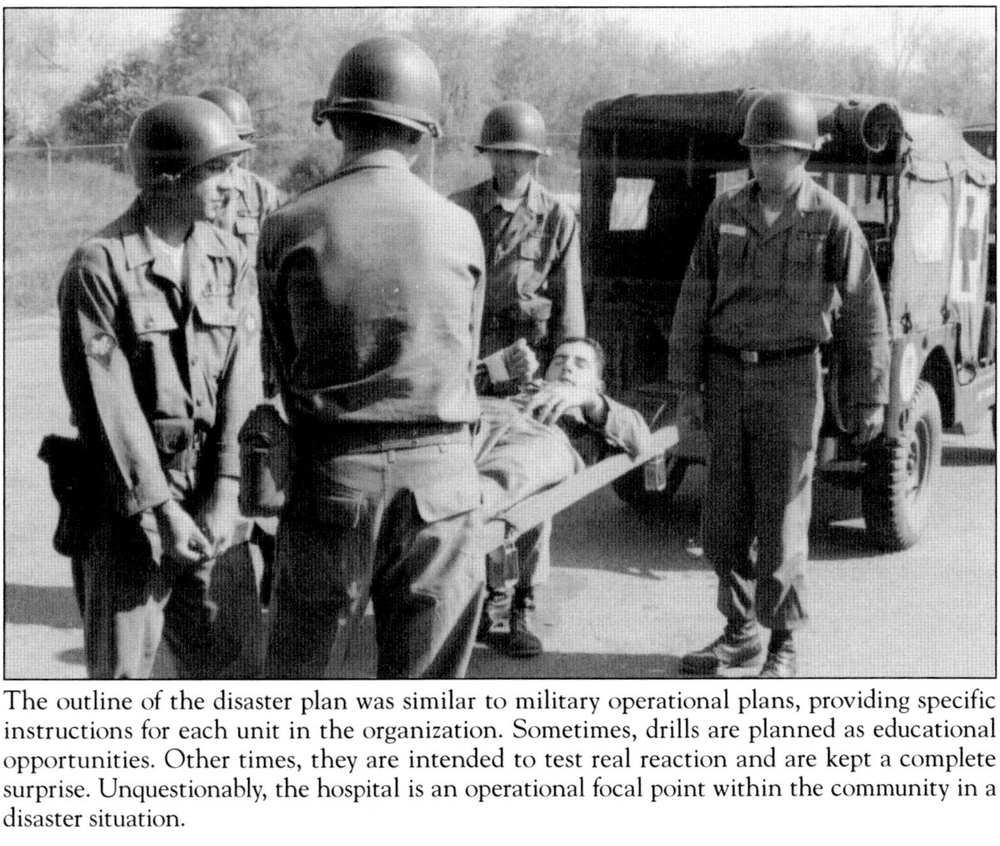

The outline of the disaster plan was similar to military operational plans, providing specific instructions for each unit in the organization. Sometimes, drills are planned as educational opportunities. Other times, they are intended to test real reaction and are kept a complete surprise. Unquestionably, the hospital is an operational focal point within the community in a disaster situation.

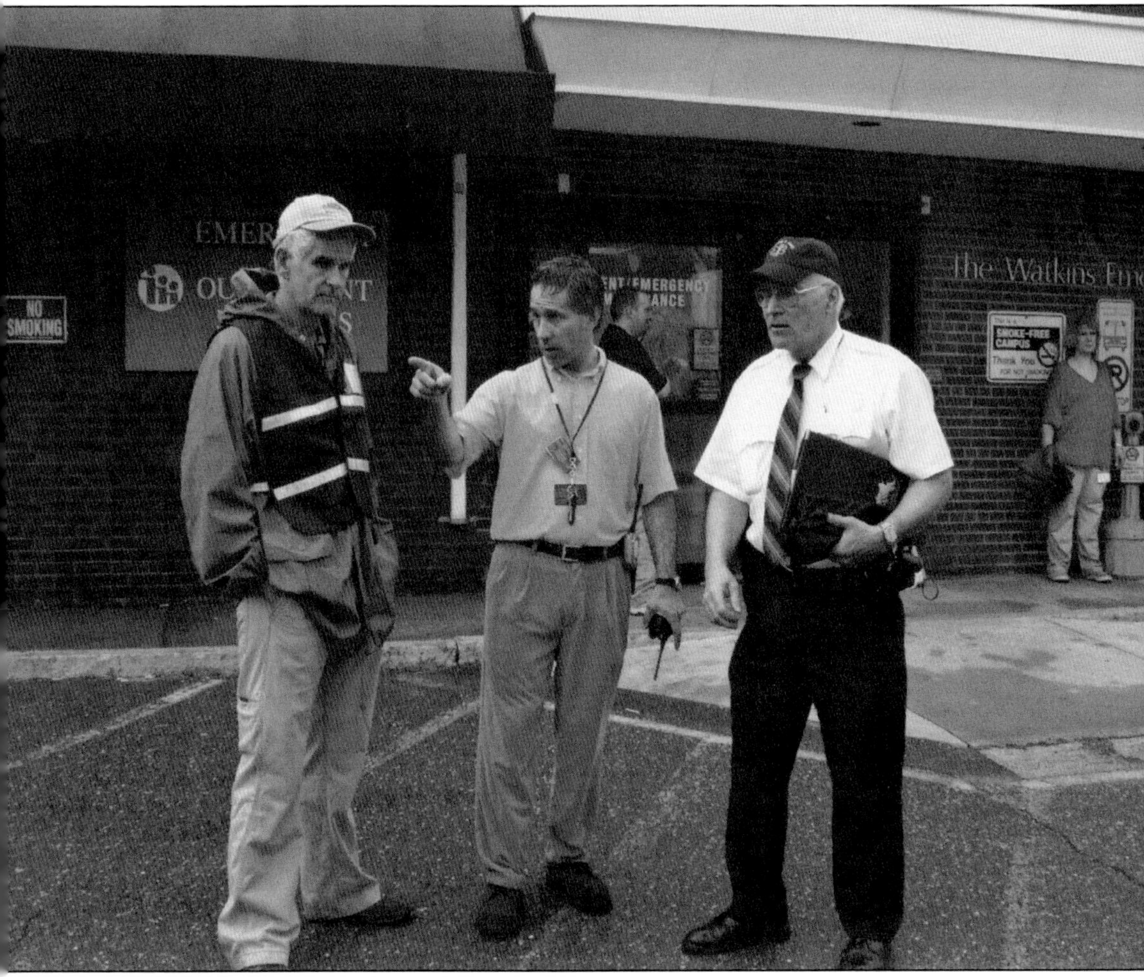

Today, all hospitals in the state of Massachusetts are required to have a disaster committee. The committee consists of administrators, physicians, nurses, and staff and is responsible for training and the coordination of disaster drills. All hospitals are required to execute two disaster drills per year. Because of the enormous amount of planning and preparation necessary to execute a drill, this committee meets at least once per month. There is also a regional meeting once a month. In this photograph, a disaster drill is underway. From left to right are Bernie Sullivan (from the Gardner Board of Health), Scott Janssens (Heywood Hospital's disaster drill team leader), and Jim Wood (owner of Wood's Ambulance in Gardner). Incidentally, Janssens remembers when Boy Scouts were used as victims in a disaster drill in 1973. The simulated disaster occurred at the Gardner Fish and Gun Club. As a participant, Janssens recalls being slathered in makeup to mimic wounds. His mock injury was an arm fracture. He was transported to the armory where the lightly injured were being treated.

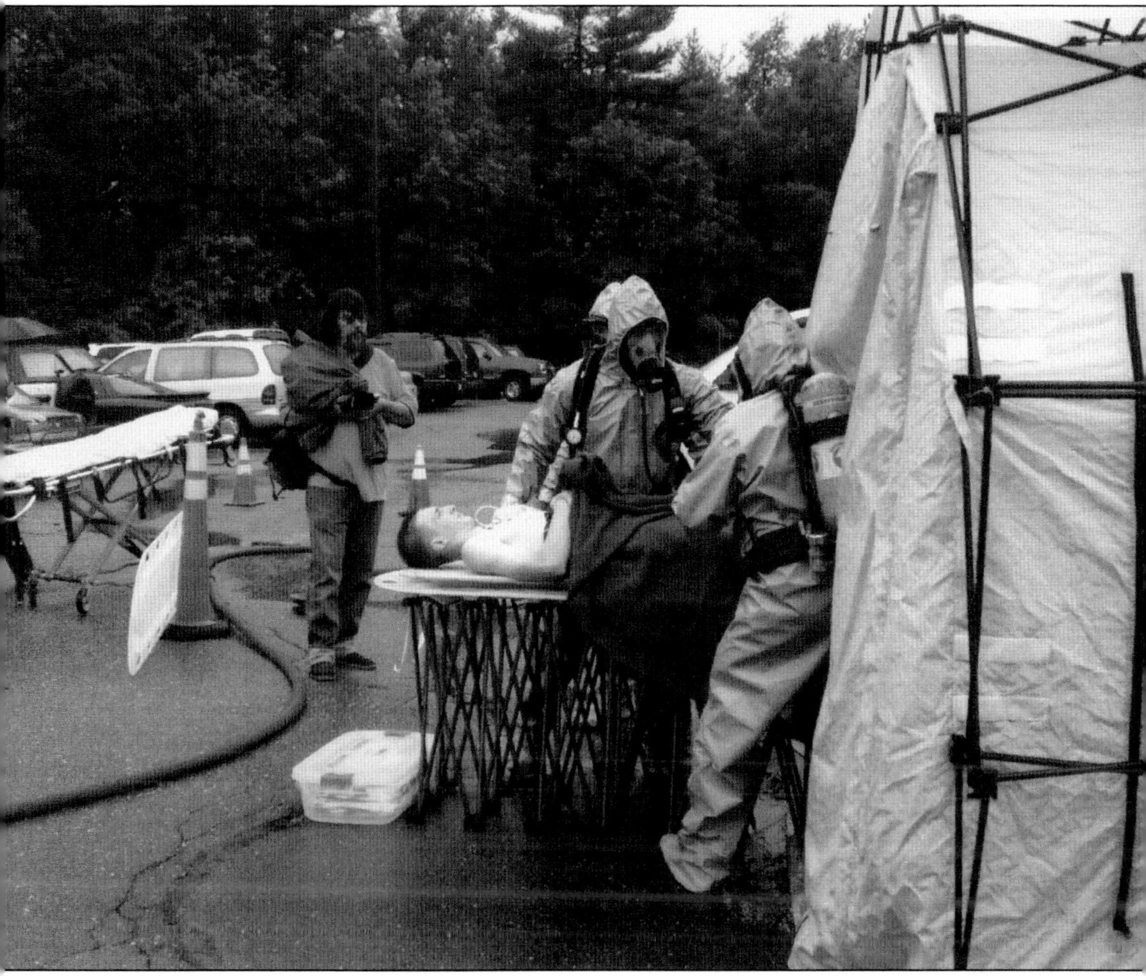

This is a hazardous material (HazMat) disaster drill for practicing mass decontamination. Involved are the police department and all the local fire departments. Using grant money, the state purchased a decontamination tent for every hospital in Massachusetts with an emergency department. The tent is like a human car wash. It has three sections: one each for males and females and a section for stretchers. There are four more sections within each of those. The first section is for disrobing. The contaminated clothes are passed out to a firefighter who marks and stores them. The subject then walks through showerheads that spray warm water and soap. Next is an area used to dry off with towels. Lastly, the subject is redressed in either another set of street clothes or a hazardous material suit. The state hazardous material team says that 99 percent of contamination is on shoes and clothes. The tent is completely self-contained. It has a generator for power and a heater for water. It needs only a water source. It takes 45 minutes to set up and costs $64,000.

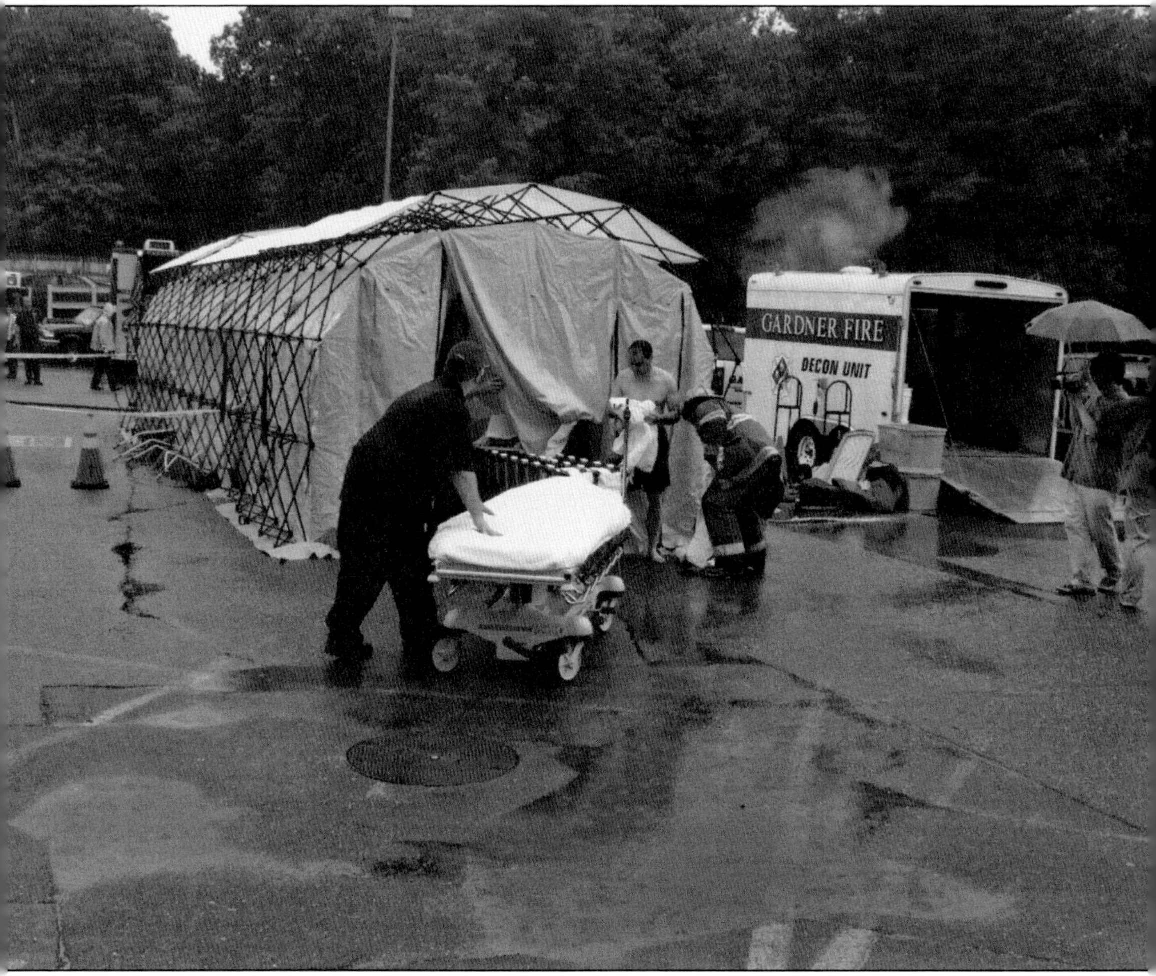

Heywood Hospital's decontamination tent is housed at the Gardner Fire Department (GFD). Additionally, every fire district has one. In an event of six people or less, the tent is not accessed. The hospital would conduct its own decontamination assisted by the GFD. The hospital's new emergency room is equipped with a two-person decontamination room. Interestingly, the manufacturer of the tents came to Massachusetts to market them. After evaluation, the state's hazardous material staff agreed to purchase significant numbers if certain changes were made to the design. The manufacturer now makes the Massachusetts Protocol (MP) tent. They are sold worldwide with the exception of England. Because of sensitivities regarding a connection to the colonies—especially Massachusetts—England purchases the same design under the name Her Majesty's Tent. Recently, the ice storm of 2008 was a huge disaster for the area. Some were without power, water, or communication for weeks. Local hospitals were fiercely challenged by the necessity to respond to the needs of area residents. Unwaveringly, Heywood Hospital's disaster team rose to each challenge as it presented itself.

Seven

Growing with the Community

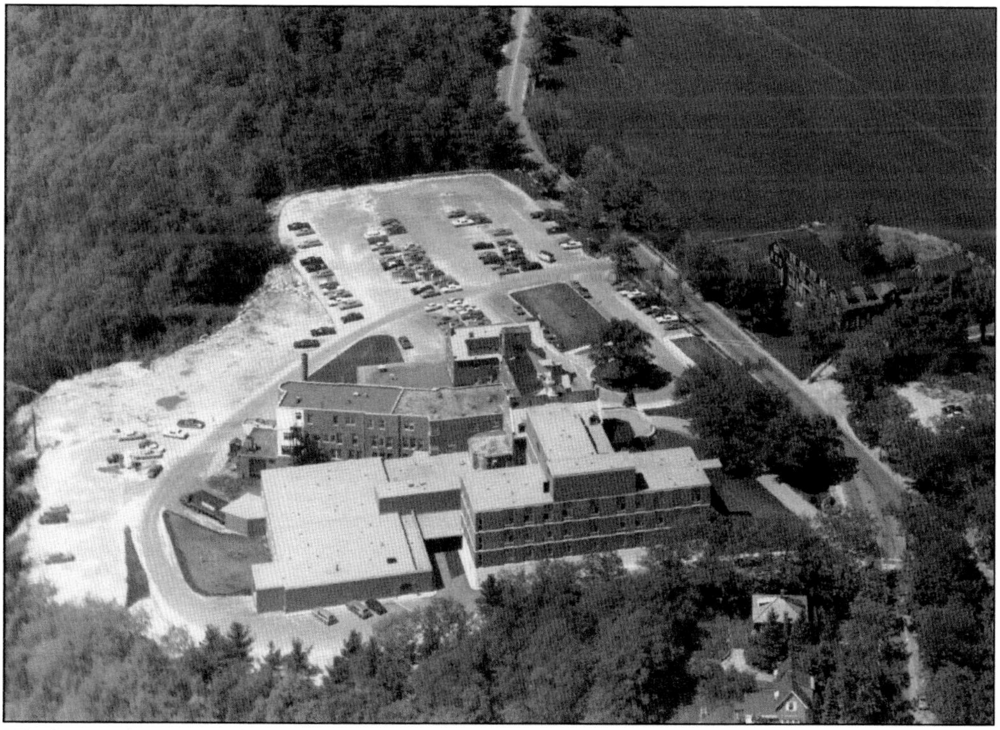

The hospital continued to grow, providing new and improved services to the community. In 1971, a food service with kitchen and cafeteria were added to the southwest side of Heywood Hospital adjacent to the emergency department. With a capacity of 156 people, the dining room serves 800 meals per day to patients, staff, and townspeople who enjoy the excellent cuisine and a scenic view of Crystal Lake beyond the trees.

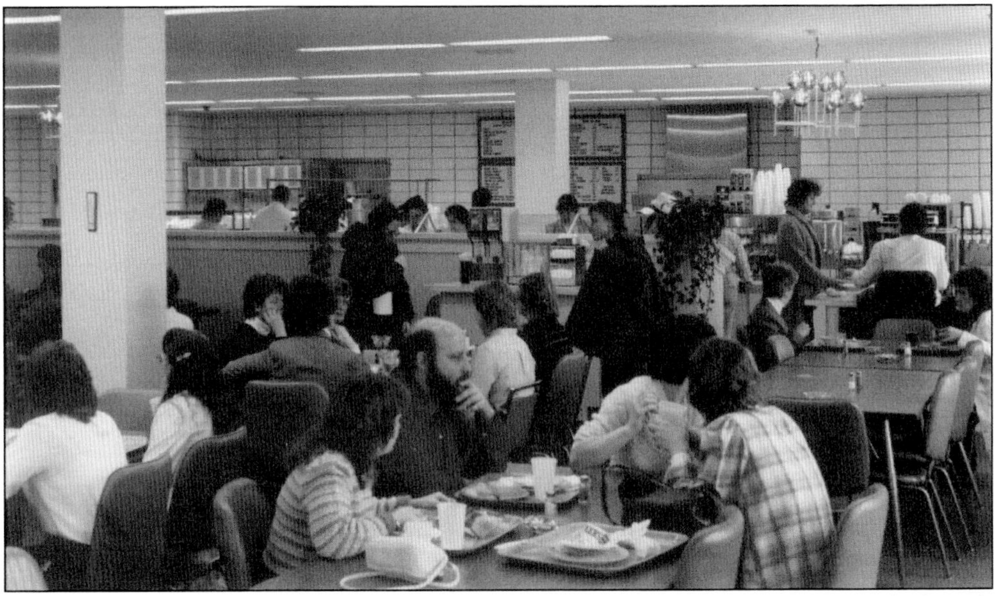

Hospital employees and local residents enjoy their meals and conversation while others file through the cafeteria line in the background. The dining room can also be divided in half and used as conference space, providing two conference rooms. During the ice storm of 2008, Heywood Hospital provided 1,900 meals, most of them free of charge, to the townspeople and staff members over a 24-hour period. Serving breakfast, lunch, dinner, and breakfast the following morning, Heywood Hospital provided for the many people in the community who were in need during this disaster. In the image below, the kitchen crew is hard at work preparing meals not only for the cafeteria, but also for the patients at Heywood Hospital.

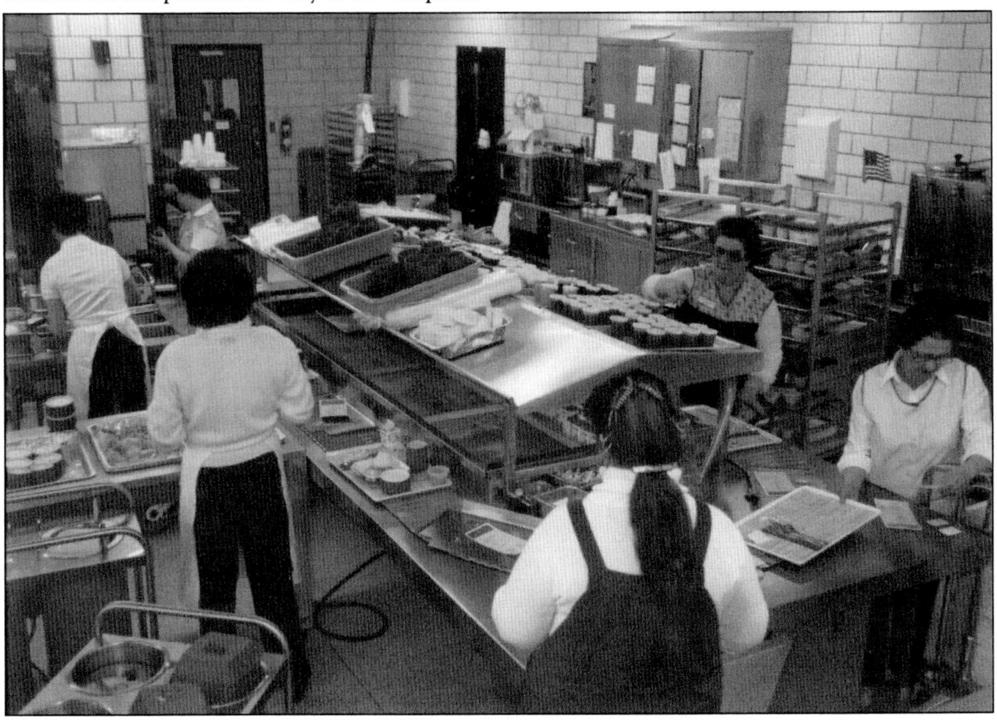

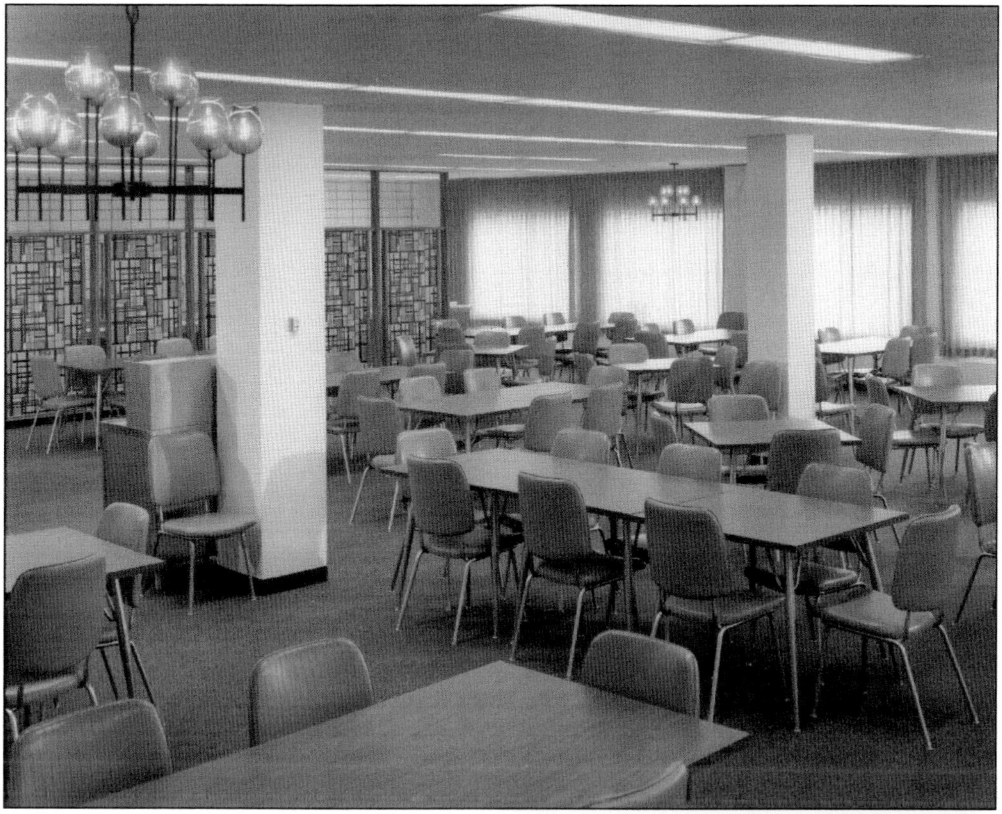

As evidenced by the lighting fixtures and wall treatment, the new decor was certainly reflective of the era. Yellows and oranges were the color scheme. Furniture and decorations have been updated at least twice since 1978. No one was prouder of the food service facilities than Harold Callahan, the first CEO of Heywood Hospital. Previous administrators had been registered nurse supervisors. A joyful Irishman with great administrative skills, he not only oversaw this addition, but also the Favor Wing and new emergency room. Coming to Heywood Hospital from Dartmouth-Hitchcock Hospital in New Hampshire, Callahan was CEO from 1953 to 1975.

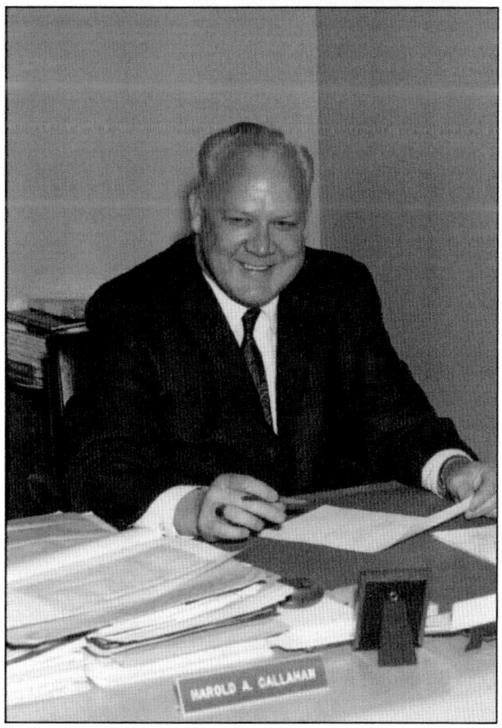

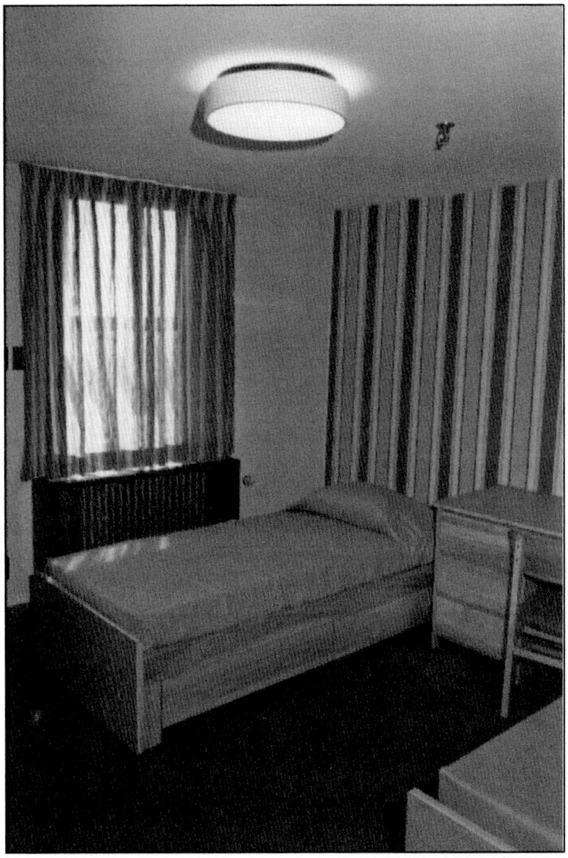

The closing of the East Gardner State Hospital in 1953 created a need to serve the mentally ill in the Gardner area. In 1977, Dr. David Gill began setting up psychiatric services at Heywood Hospital. The third floor of the North Wing was renovated, and the mental health unit (MHU) opened its doors to patients in 1978. Gill has been the chief of psychiatric services since its inception. The unit cares for acutely ill patients aged 16 and up, and is licensed for 12 beds. The MHU at Heywood Hospital has been recognized by the Massachusetts Department of Mental Health and other organizations as a "best practice" site. Excellent outcomes include a lower than average length of stay and fewer patients needing readmittance for further treatment. These images from 1978 show a patient's room and a lounge.

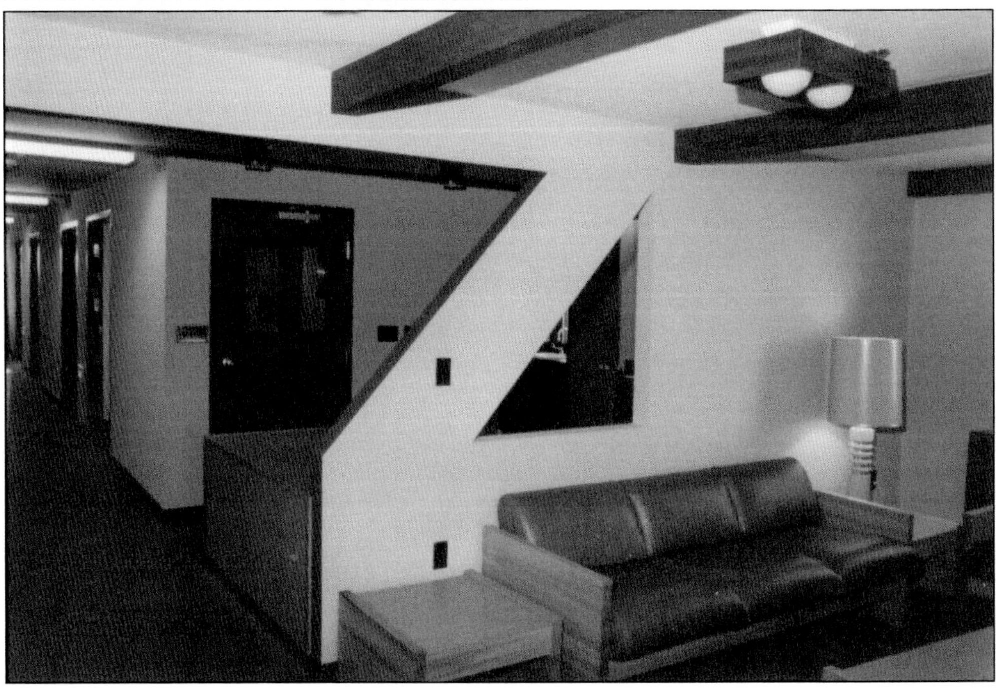

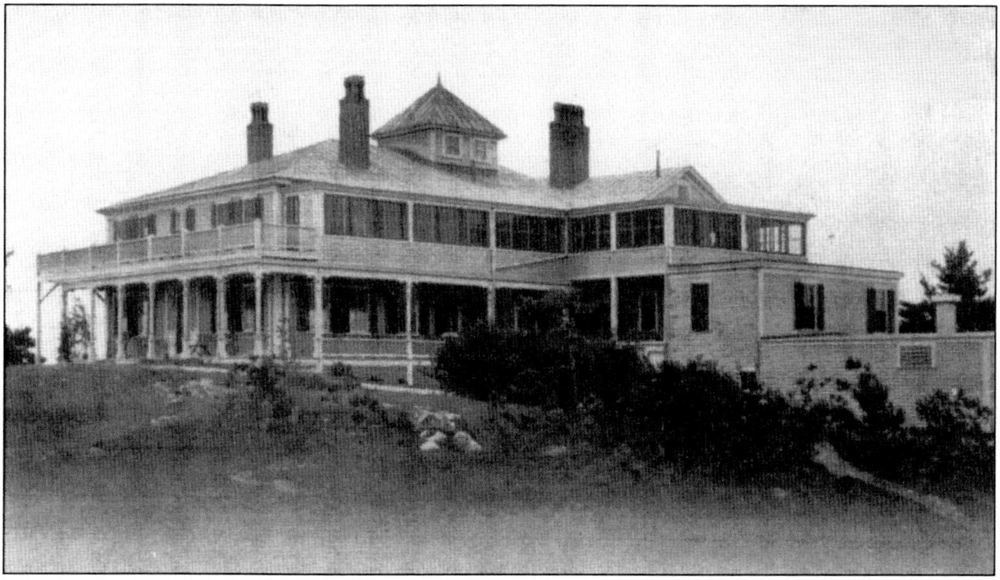

The nearby town of Winchendon, Massachusetts, began providing medical care to its residents with the establishment of the Millers River Hospital in 1907. Incorporating as the Winchendon Hospital in 1927, it continued to serve its residents at this site until moving its operation to the old "Town Farm" property in 1948. Pictured above in that new location, the Winchendon Hospital had a license for 30 beds. Additions were made in the 1960s, but changes to public health regulations for small hospitals throughout the 1970s made its independent operation difficult to maintain. In 1982, the Winchendon Hospital became affiliated with Heywood Hospital and was renamed the Winchendon Health Center (below). (Above, courtesy of WHS.)

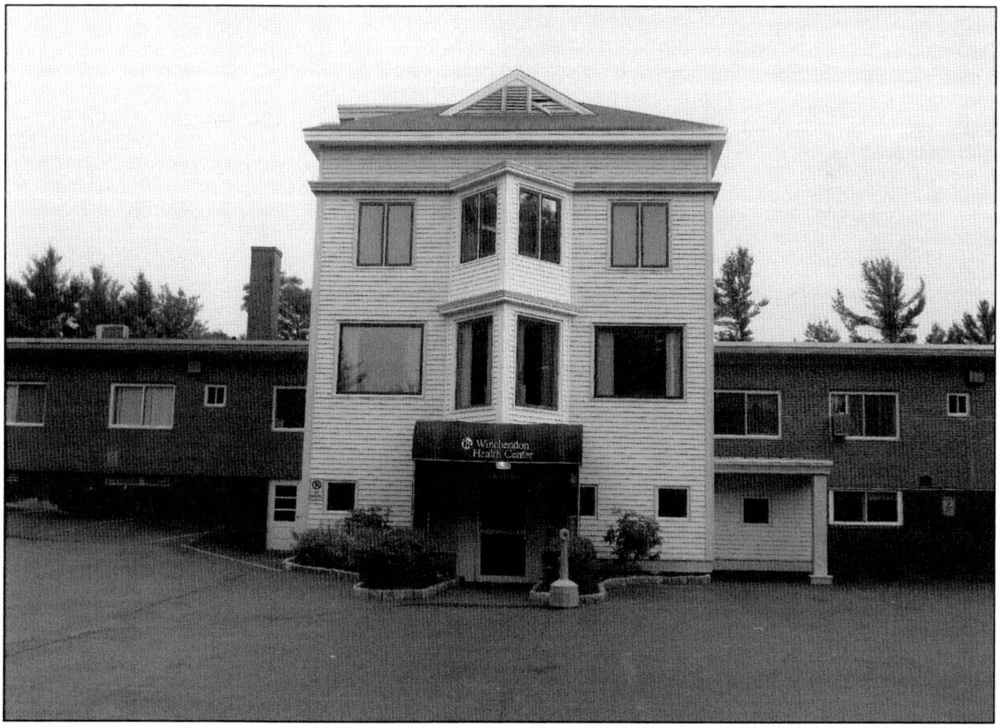

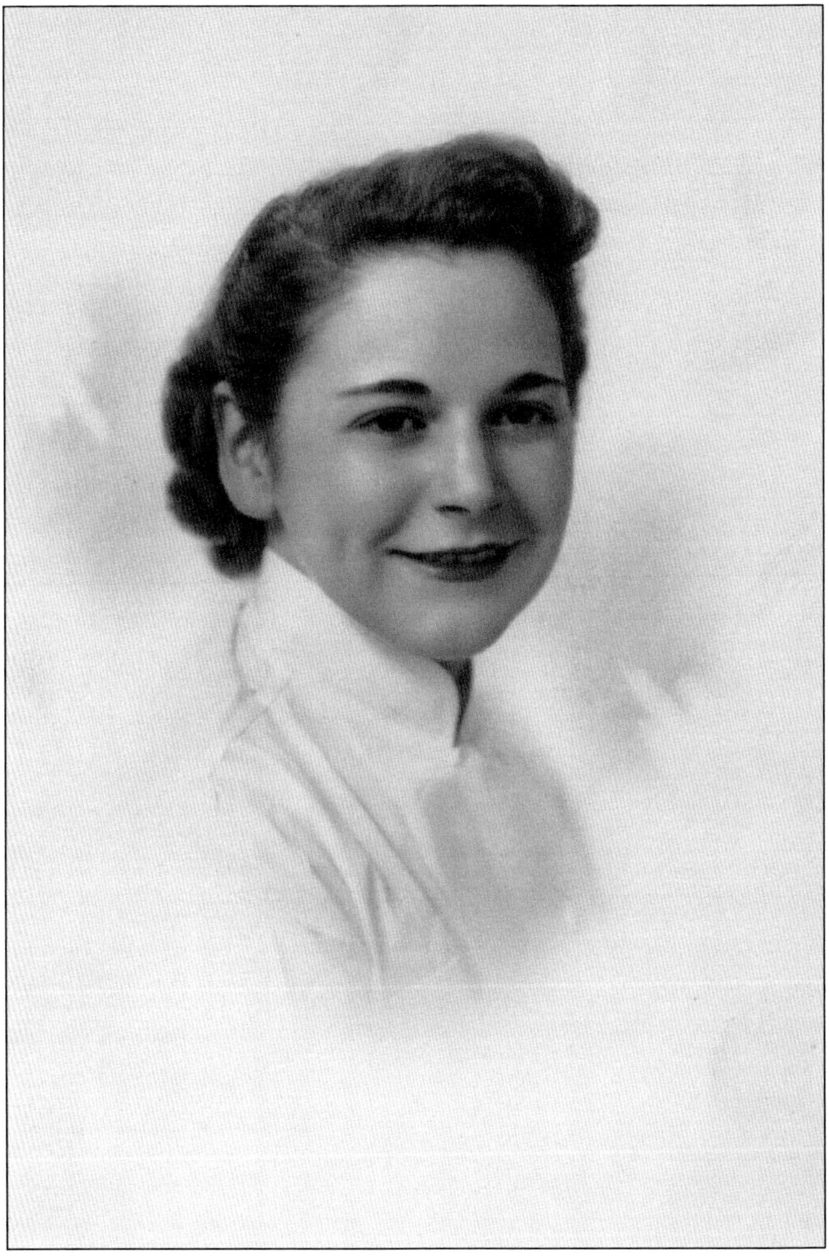

The Winchendon Health Center is an outpatient, Heywood Hospital satellite facility operating as a family practice health center. Its mission is to provide outpatient care for the residents of Winchendon and surrounding communities. Mary Ann Lemire Gandy, a Winchendon native, was an X-ray technician and supervisor at Winchendon Hospital in the early 1950s and continued her employment there long after it became affiliated with Heywood Hospital and converted to the Winchendon Health Center. In the mid-1950s, X-ray technicians from Massachusetts General Hospital were sent to observe Gandy. Intrigued by an X-ray brought to them by a patient sent for further evaluation, they were to observe the settings she used to attain such an accurate "butterfly view" of the patient's sinuses. Apparently, Gandy's technique utilized a certain angle through the back of the skull not yet routinely done elsewhere. (Courtesy of Edward J. Gandy.)

There was a hospital high on a hill. It served a small town and it did it well. It grew and thrived and glowed like a star. And the patients came from near and far.

We had Surgery, Maternity and Pedi too, and cared for the ill and elderly, who stayed for 5 years or only a day, and nobody questioned or wanted a say.

The Lab and X-ray departments grew. We added two wings, complaints were few. We had our laughs and we had our tears, but we did our work well for all the years.

Our patients were pleasant, as a whole, except for that "ornery goat" in 24, who refused to shave or bathe and would scold and would make you want to walk off the floor.

In "66 O.B. went out the door, no more mommies or babies to care for. No more waiting for birth, or that first cry. Is it a girl or a boy? Twins.. Oh My!

This same year we started Review, with Dr. Millard and Jeannette C., too, who looked at the charts once a week for sure to decide if admissions were acute or the patient was here on a "toot"= R&R.

In 1970 with State Inspection, we closed out Pedi with much trepidation. The State said "no kids can be kept", without a "Chief of Pediatrics".

In this same year the Feds came along and said let's take a look at what's going on. At all this money being spent for hospital care, "Is it worth every cent"?

Out in Chicago we heard from some "birds" who wanted to come here and be heard. For $500 we'll come in for review, we'll tell you your problems and corrections too, and present you a plaque for your wall in the hall we thought at this time that this might be a "ball".

Reviews became costly as years went by, from $500 to $2200 in '79. The team went from two up to four and they started to make us measure "doors". We went upstairs and downstairs, outdoors and in, and we learned about "siamese couplings" and other things.

In '75 PSRO wanted a voice and it appeared to all we had little choice. Standards were placed on us day after day and we had less and less to say. Questions were asked "is this acute care?", "How long do you plan for this patient to stay"? "A letter will be sent without delay."

Plan after plan were made for this plot and then they decided to buy another lot, to do what they planned for up on the hill, but found they couldn't meet the bill. We argued in Boston to save our "fate" but nothing has worked up to date, and we often times wonder, is it to late?

And here it is Dec. "81, a time for remembering and celebrations. We've lost good friends over the years, you know who I mean, but please no tears. New friends, new faces have come along, to fill the spaces of friends long gone.

There was a hospital high on the hill, it served a small town and it did it well.

This untitled poem reminiscing about Winchendon Hospital was penned by Gandy in December 1981. It is a bittersweet account chronicling the hospital's growth and successes, followed by some of the various regulations and reviews imposed by outside organizations that contributed to the eventual closure of the institution. Gandy retired from the Winchendon Health Center in the late 1980s after 34 years of service. Incidentally, Gandy's husband, Edward J. Gandy, is one of the last surviving members of the submarine crew that rescued US Navy pilot George H.W. Bush from the sea when his plane was shot down in the Pacific Ocean by Japanese aircraft during World War II. He still resides in Winchendon, Massachusetts. President Bush, forever grateful, continues to host an annual summer cookout at his compound on Walker's Point to thank these men to whom he owes his life. (Courtesy of Edward J. Gandy.)

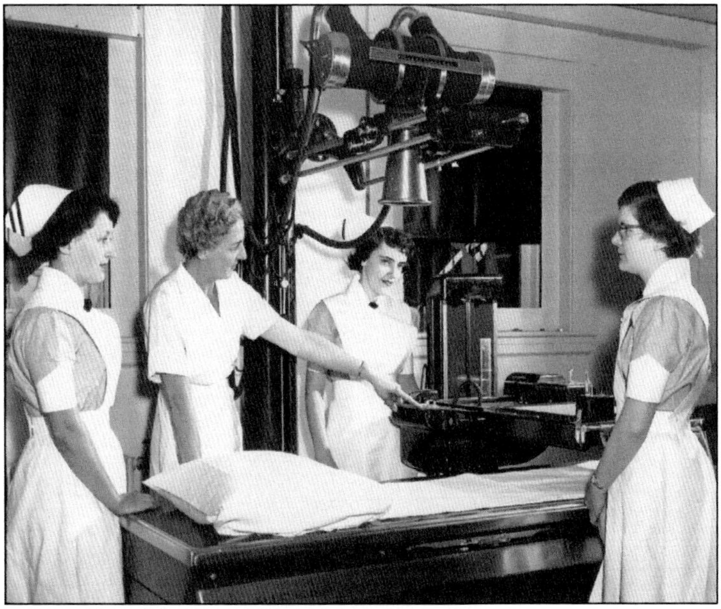

Wilhelm Rontgen invented the first X-ray machine in 1895; hence, there is no mention of an X-ray suite in the original hospital plans. In this image, Marge Sullivan (second from left), supervisor of X-ray and laboratory, demonstrates to nursing students the use of fluoroscopy equipment whereby the radiologist can view various organs, such as the lung, heart, and stomach. Only a cone protects from excess radiation exposure.

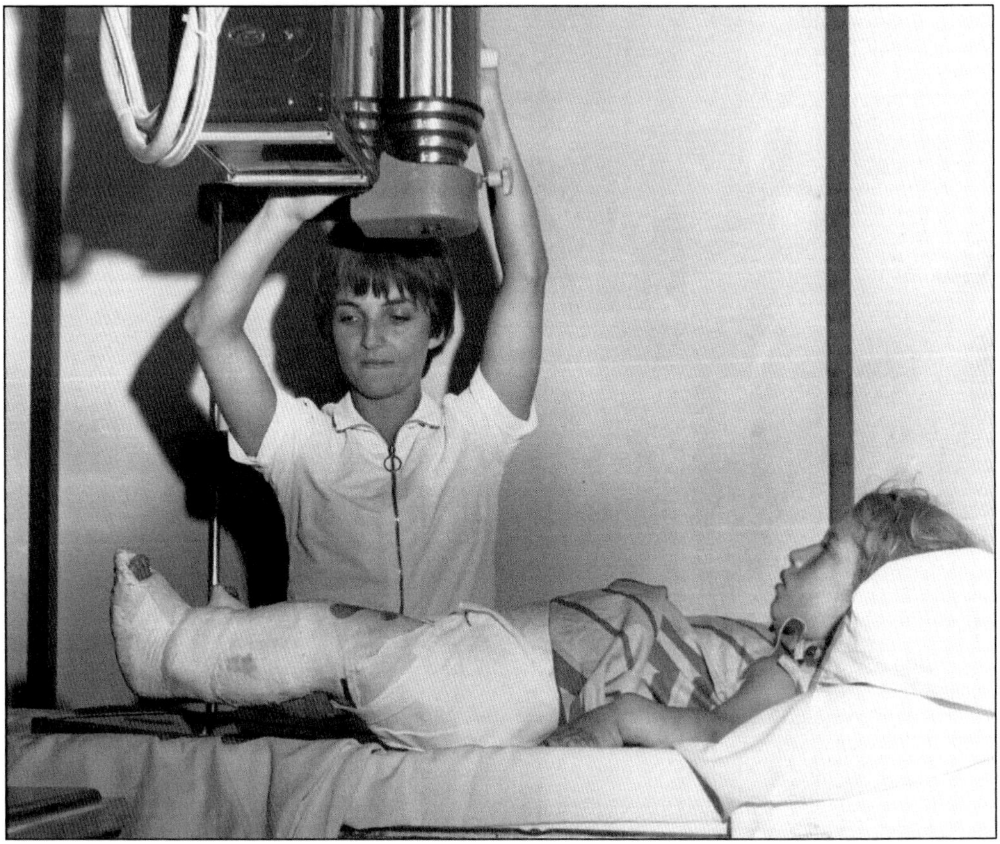

This X-ray machine does not have a cone, but instead utilizes a colometer that is able to limit the radiation exposure much better than just a cone. Radiation exposure is very important in x-raying children. Mary Nordman is x-raying the left leg of a child in a cast.

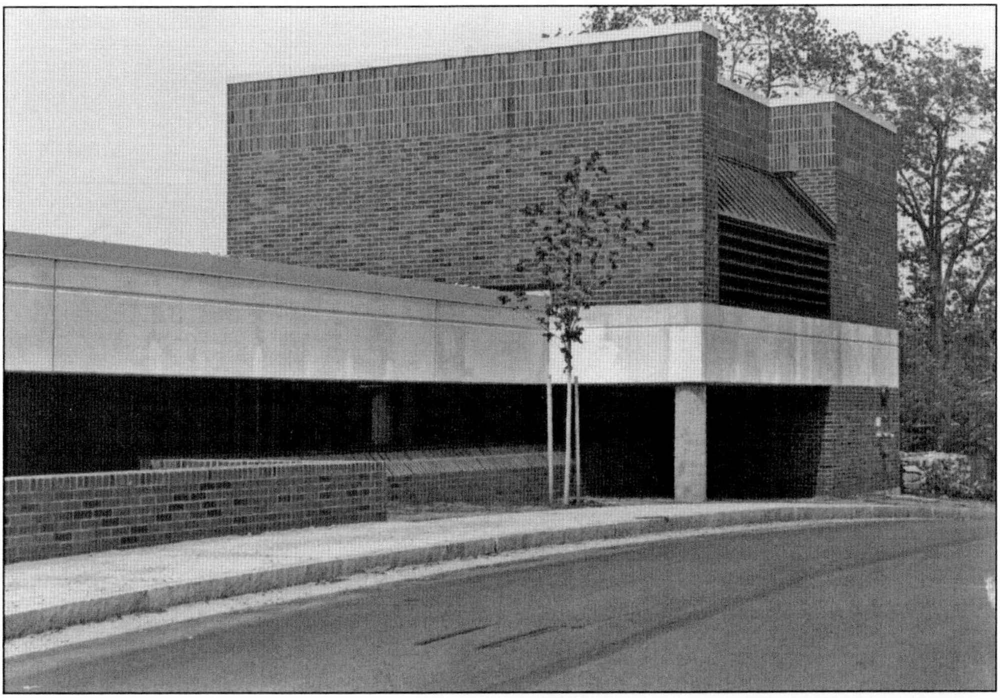

Under the guidance of chief of radiology Dr. Paul St. Aubin, a new radiology wing was built on the south side of Heywood Hospital adjacent to the Favor Wing's ground floor, which houses the surgical suite and emergency room. This provided smoother travel between the departments. The new radiology wing provided two large rooms with fluoroscopy capabilities utilizing television monitors; one of the rooms was used for angiography and radiological intervention procedures. A third room was used for ultrasound and another for nuclear scans. There were two rooms for routine X-rays and a mammogram suite. The image above shows the 1982 radiology wing. The image at right shows an early X-ray machine from the 1940s.

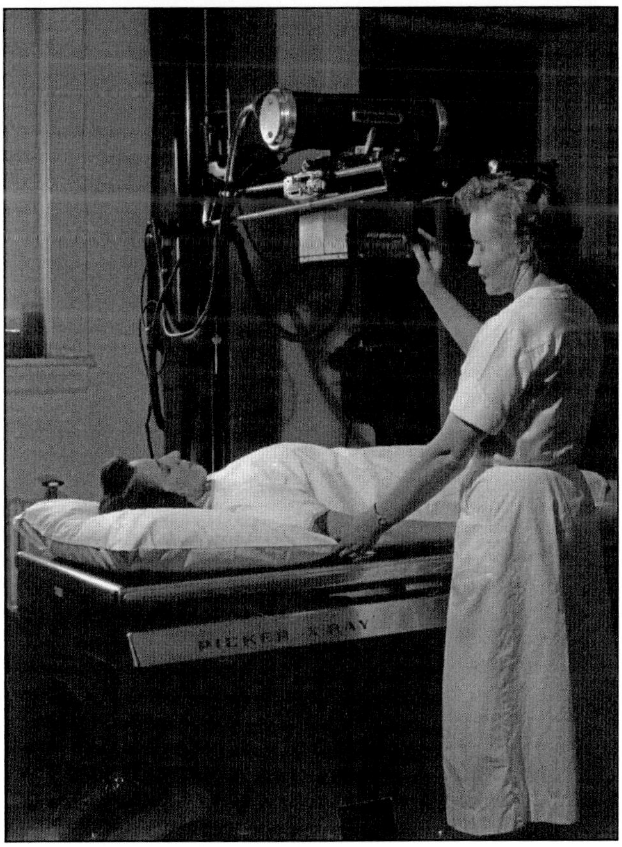

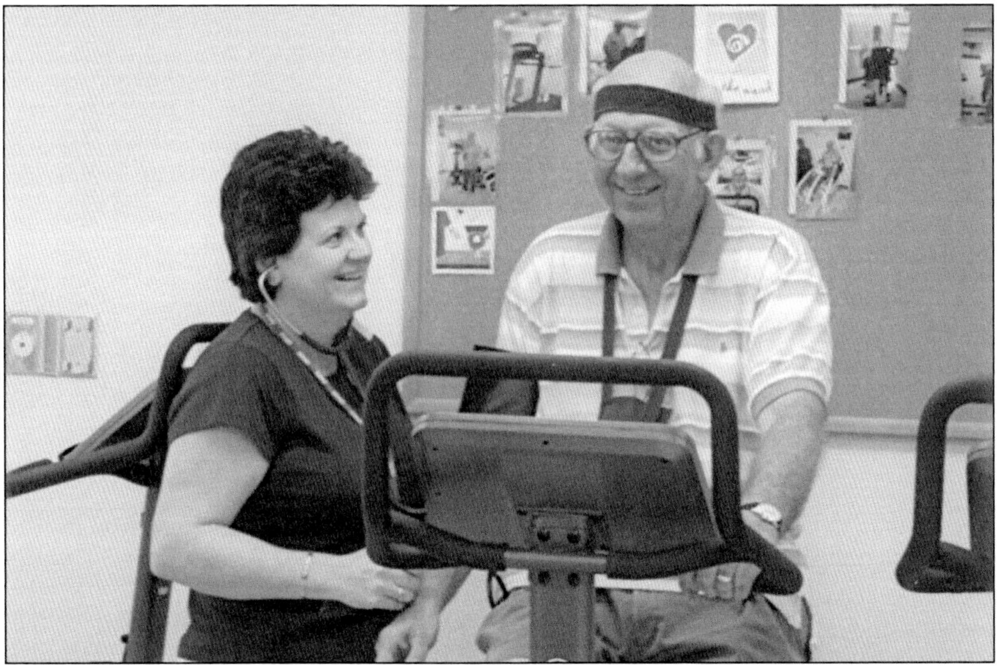

In the 1980s, Dr. Owen Christensen preached the benefits of exercise for coronary artery disease. He was impressed by the work of Dr. Paul Dudley White, renowned cardiologist at Massachusetts General Hospital. In 1986, the Heywood Cardiac Rehabilitation Center opened. Patients were given appropriate exercises while having their heart and vital signs monitored and were educated in risk factors. Manager Theresa LeBlanc closely monitors David Poliks on an exercise bicycle.

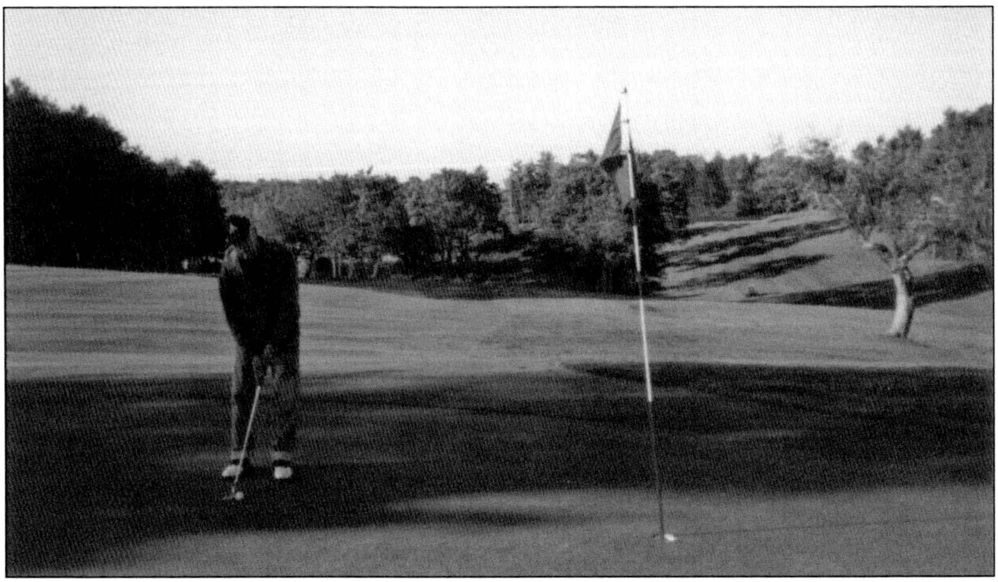

In 2004, George Billings was enjoying a round of golf at the Gardner Municipal Golf Course. At about 11:30 that morning, he collapsed from cardiac arrest on the seventh fairway. Thanks to cardiopulmonary resuscitation (CPR) and a defibrillator in the clubhouse, George survived. Cardiac rehabilitation with appropriate exercise and support helped Billings to return to golf. This image shows him playing golf in 2011, seven years after his cardiac event.

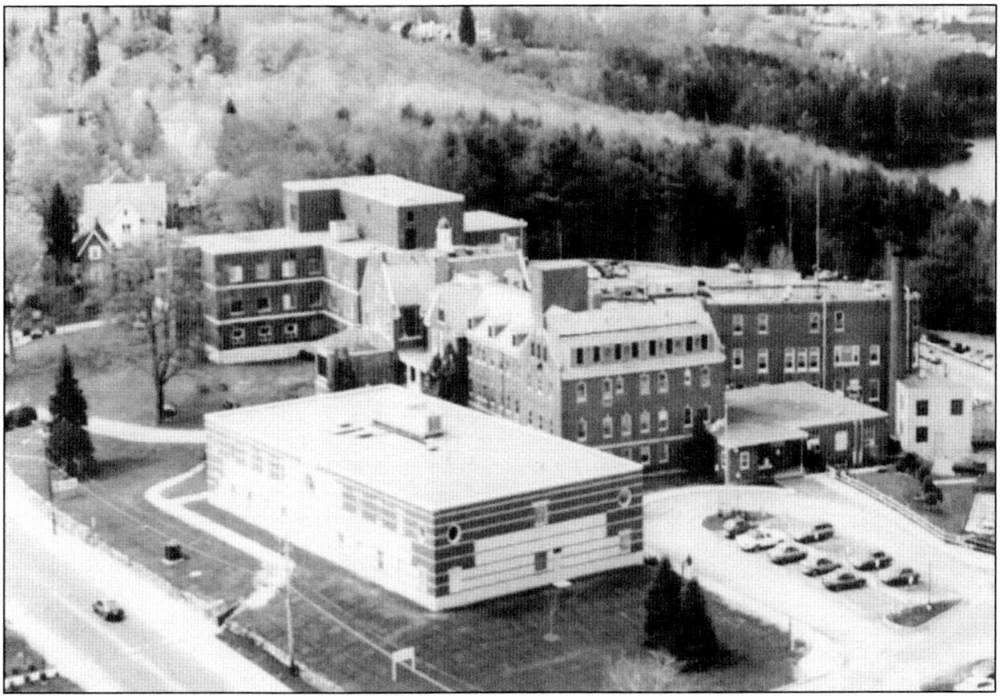

Physicians are key to providing patient care, and Heywood Hospital sought to increase its physician base in the late 1980s. A lack of office space was prohibitive in recruiting new physicians, but the hospital did not have the capital to invest in an office building. A group of eight physicians and a pharmacist provided the capital to finance the project. This image shows the original Medical Arts Building.

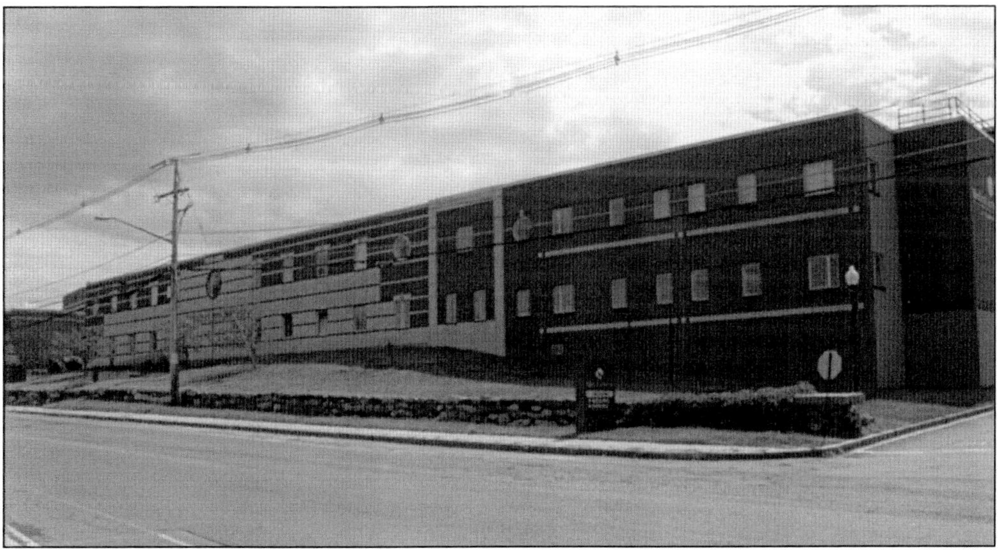

Heywood Hospital eventually bought out the original owners and built an addition in 1996 that increased the number of physicians from 13 to 33. A pharmacy was housed in the original Medical Arts Building. The total experience was a great example of how the Heywood Hospital physicians banded together to support the hospital. This image shows the combined medical office buildings.

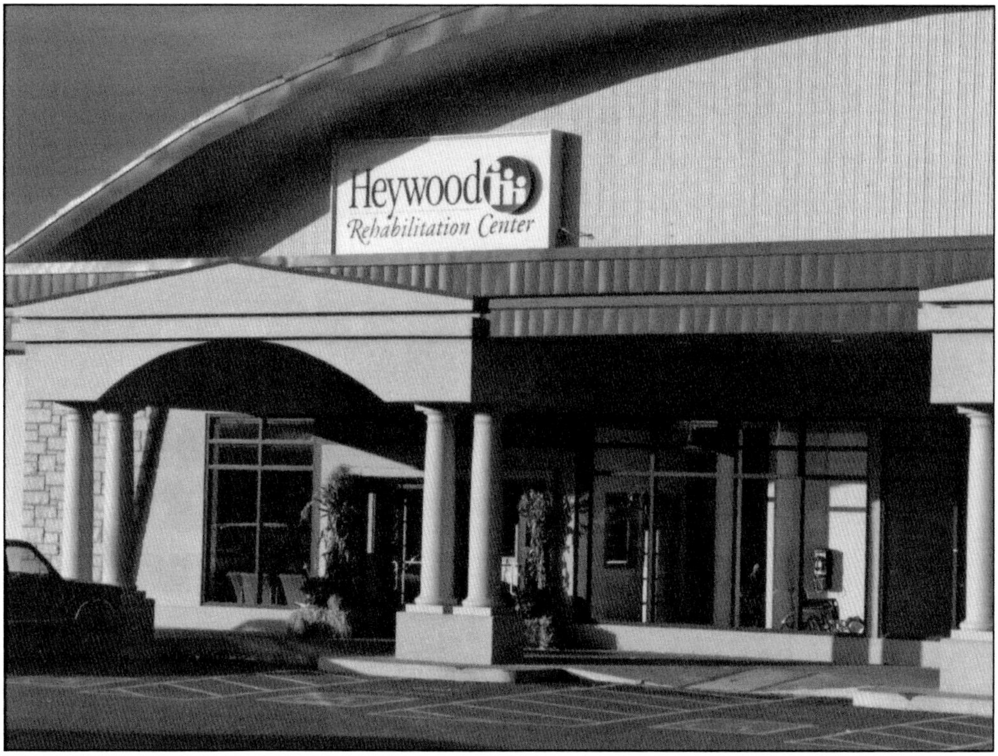

The Heywood Rehabilitation Center was relocated from Heywood Hospital to a location owned by GFA Credit Union in South Gardner. This represents an example of how a community business benefited the hospital. This not only freed up space within the hospital but also took pressure off an already congested hospital parking lot. The rehabilitation center provides not only physical therapy, but also audiology testing and treatment.

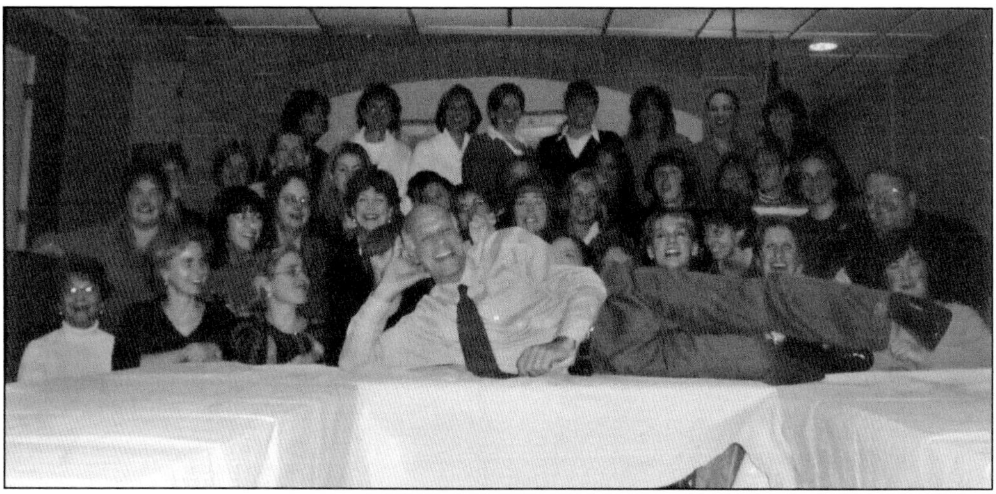

Bruce Quatrulli was the manager of the Heywood Rehabilitation Center at its inception in 1999. Quatrulli not only built the center into a multidisciplinary facility that included speech, audiology, occupational, and physical therapy services, but also exemplified the concept of teamwork within the Heywood Hospital family. This photograph shows a much-loved Quatrulli surrounded by his team. (Courtesy of Charlene Costa.)

The oncology department opened in 1986. Chief of oncology Dr. Sheila Donnelly added stability and direction to the program. Donnelly is full time at Heywood Hospital, and also works at the Dana Farber Cancer Center. This type of association has ensured the use of evidence-based practices and current treatments at a local level. Donnelly is pictured enjoying one of her favorite sports. (Courtesy of Dr. Sheila Donnelly.)

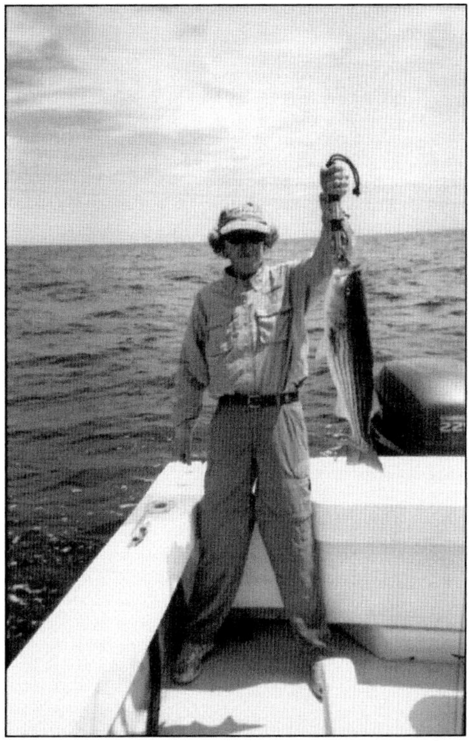

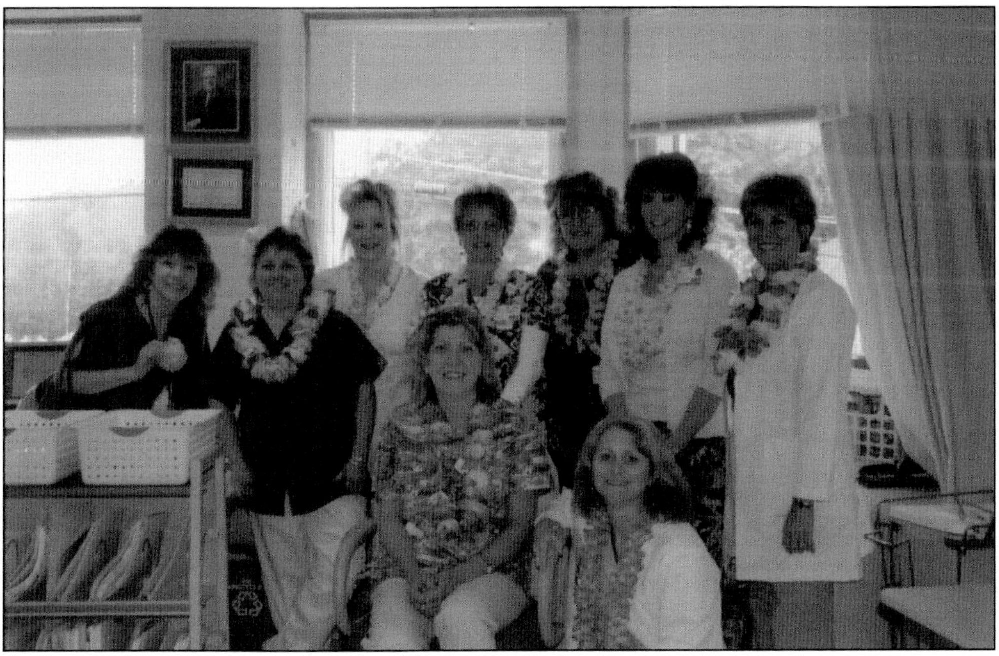

Annie Sawicki is a graduate of the Henry Heywood Memorial School of Nursing and is a well-respected retired head nurse. Preferring the traditional white nurses' uniforms with cap and pin, Sawicki often lamented the modern colorful nurses' outfits. In honor of Sawicki, the oncology personnel one day changed into all whites. Here, the oncology crew is dressed in Hawaiian garb for a Hospital Week celebration.

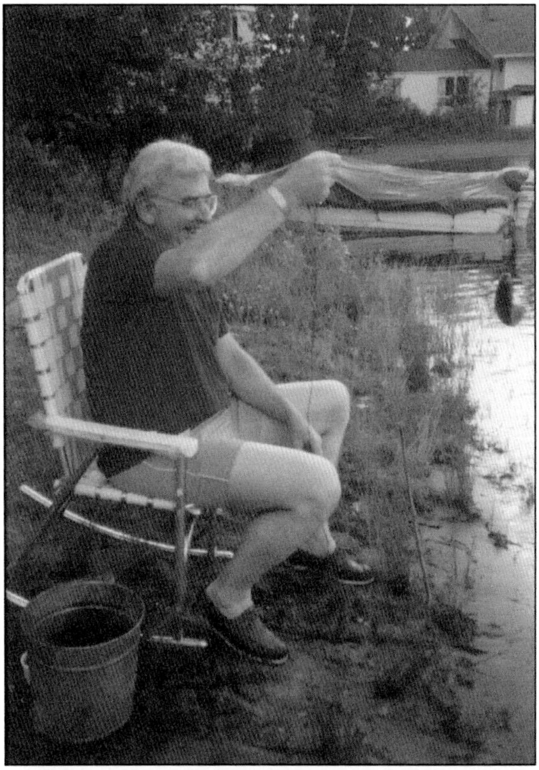

In 2001, an oncology unit was built consisting of a bay room with six chemotherapy chairs, plus private exam and treatment rooms where expert compassionate care is provided. It is named for 20-year cancer survivor Edward "Satch" Stromski. He served as chairman of the board of trustees for eight years, during which Heywood Hospital had a significant financial turnaround. A close look reveals Stromski's tiny catch. (Courtesy of Ed Stromski.)

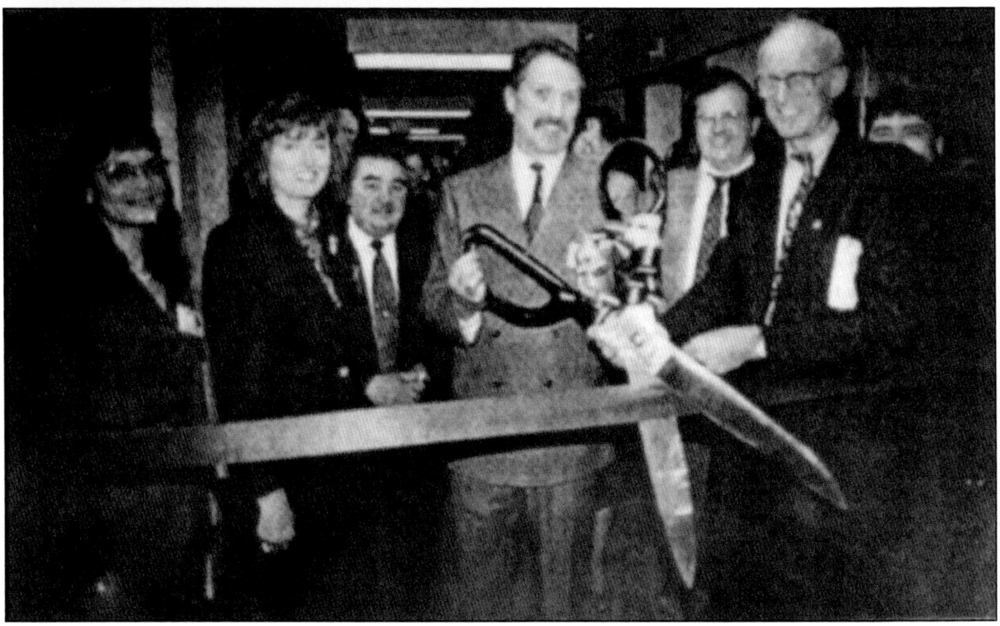

In 1995, the former pediatric floor on the West Wing was converted to the Transitional Care Center (TCC.) The 19-bed center underwent four months of renovation at a cost of $720,000. Here at the ribbon-cutting ceremony are, from left to right, director of nursing Susan Matuszewski, administrator Carol Singh, Mayor Charles Manca, CEO and president Daniel Moen, medical director John Harrington, and Rep. John Olver. (Courtesy of the *Gardner News.*)

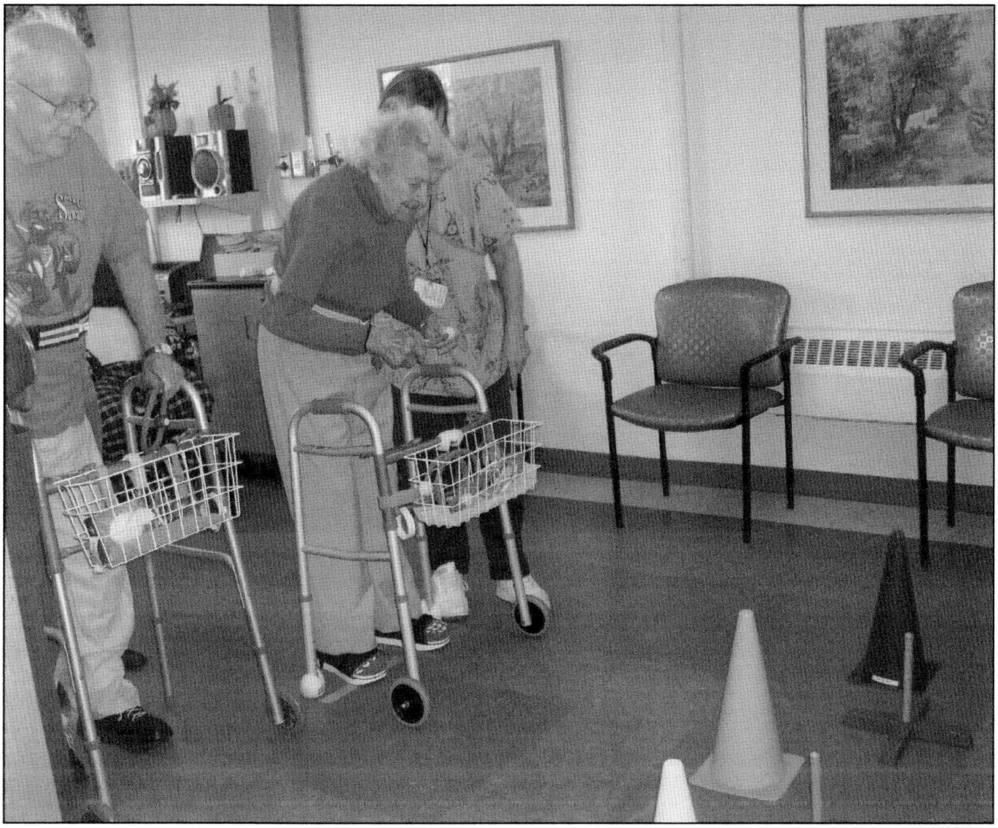

The center is designed to accept patients from the hospital who need additional medical or physical therapy treatment prior to being discharged. Heywood Hospital's TCC celebrated 14 consecutive deficiency-free surveys by the Massachusetts Department of Public Health in 2011 and was featured in 2010 in *US News and World Report* for its excellence. Above, an activities director interacts with patients. Named for Edward G. Watkins, the Watkins Emergency Center opened in 1993. Located on the ground floor of the Favor Wing, the previous emergency room had four exam rooms. The new emergency center had 10 exam rooms, X-ray facilities, and two large rooms (like the one at right) for acute problems, such as heart attacks and severe injuries. There was a separate ambulance entrance, waiting room with triage, and registration booths.

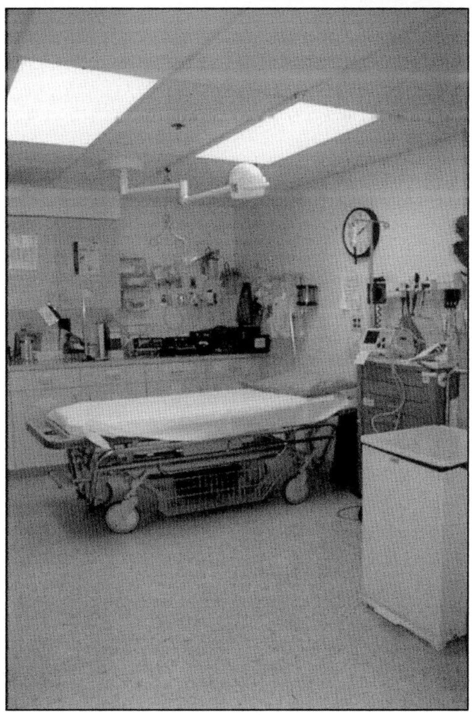

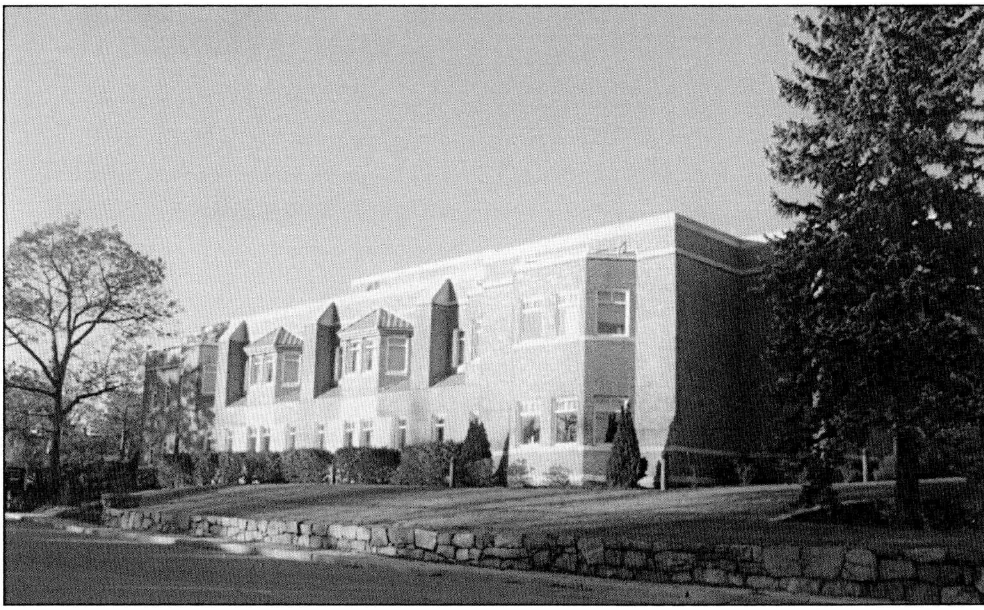

This is a two-story medical building located on the south-east side of the Heywood Hospital complex. Built in 2001, the first floor of the building houses the Thomas P. Kelly Ambulatory Care Center and the Edward I. Stromski Oncology Unit. The second floor houses the LaChance Maternity Center.

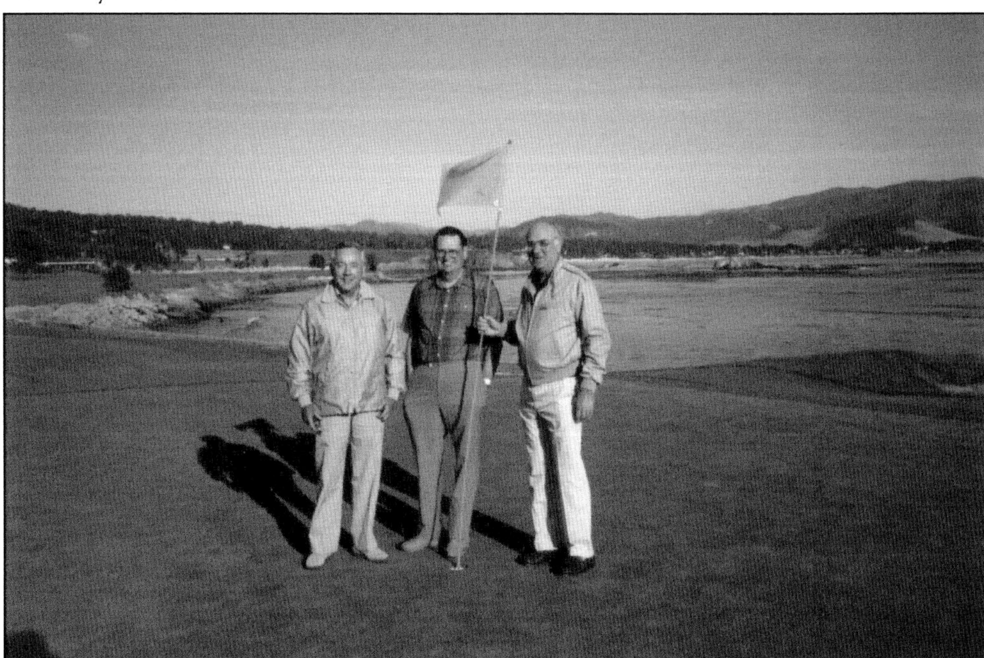

Thomas P. Kelly headed the Lilly Chemical Company in Templeton, Massachusetts, which produced paints and stains for the local furniture factories. Kelly served for a number of years on the board of trustees. A community-minded philanthropist, he was also the cochairman of the Caring for the Future campaign and cofounder of the Heywood Golf Classic. Here, Kelly (left) stands on the 18th hole at Pebble Beach with golf buddies Jim Faust (center) and Joe Rome.

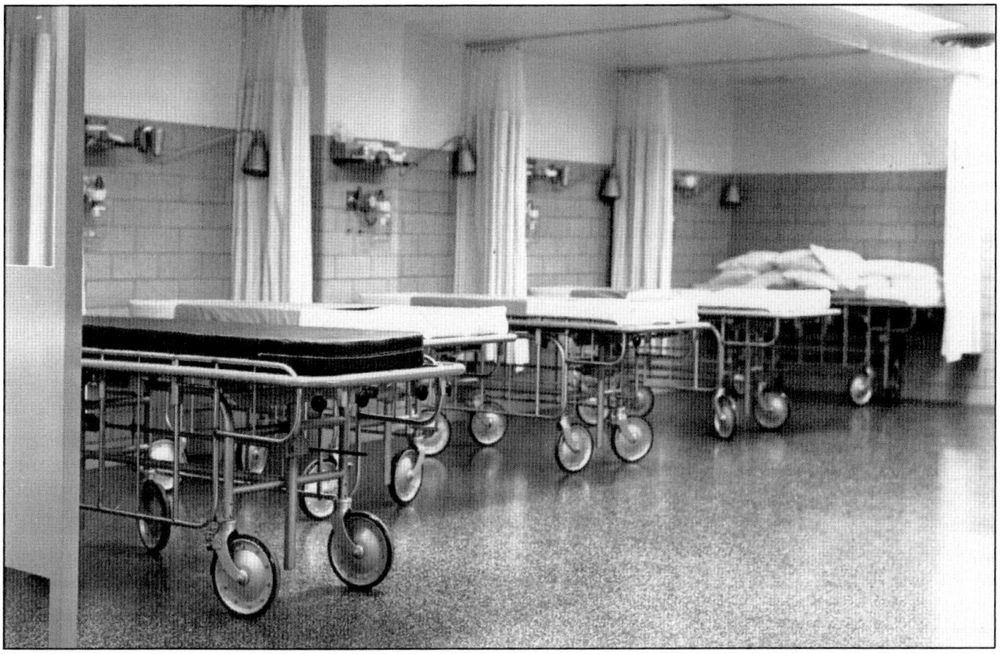

The Ambulatory Care Center is attached to the surgical suite in the Favor Wing, which facilitates the surgical day care unit. Increasingly, surgical procedures are being performed as outpatient surgery. To provide high quality postsurgical and anesthesia care, a new surgical recovery room was added. This image shows the original 1960 recovery room.

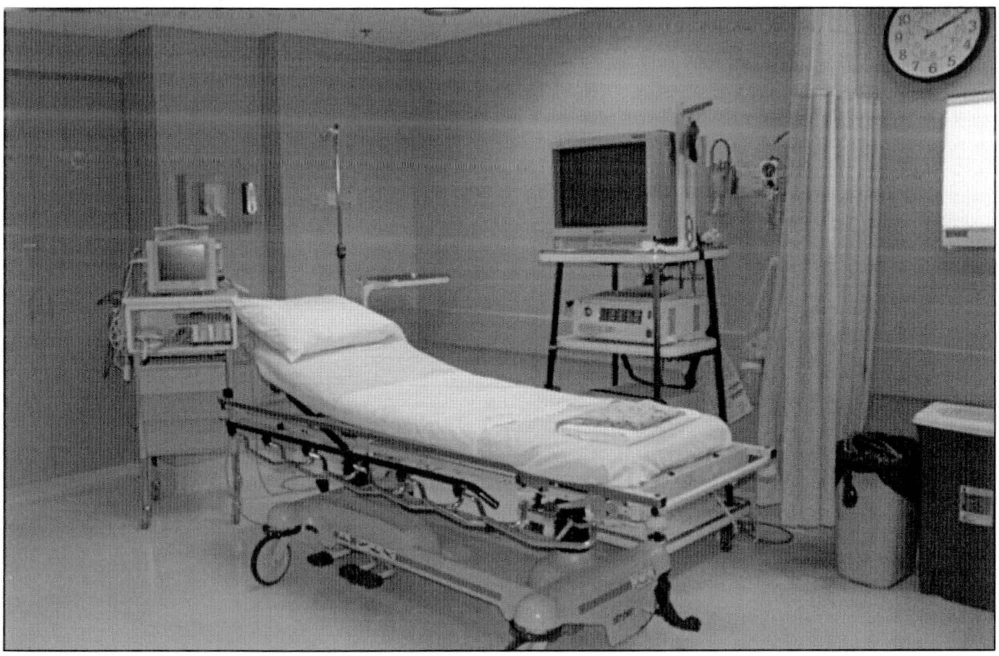

Special Procedures is located in the Ambulatory Care Center. Endoscopy, including screening for colorectal cancer via colonoscopy, is a very important procedure in today's medical care as a deterrent to cancer. Gastroscopy is utilized to visualize the esophagus and stomach for ulcers, cancer, and sources of bleeding. Shown here is an endoscopy unit and monitors.

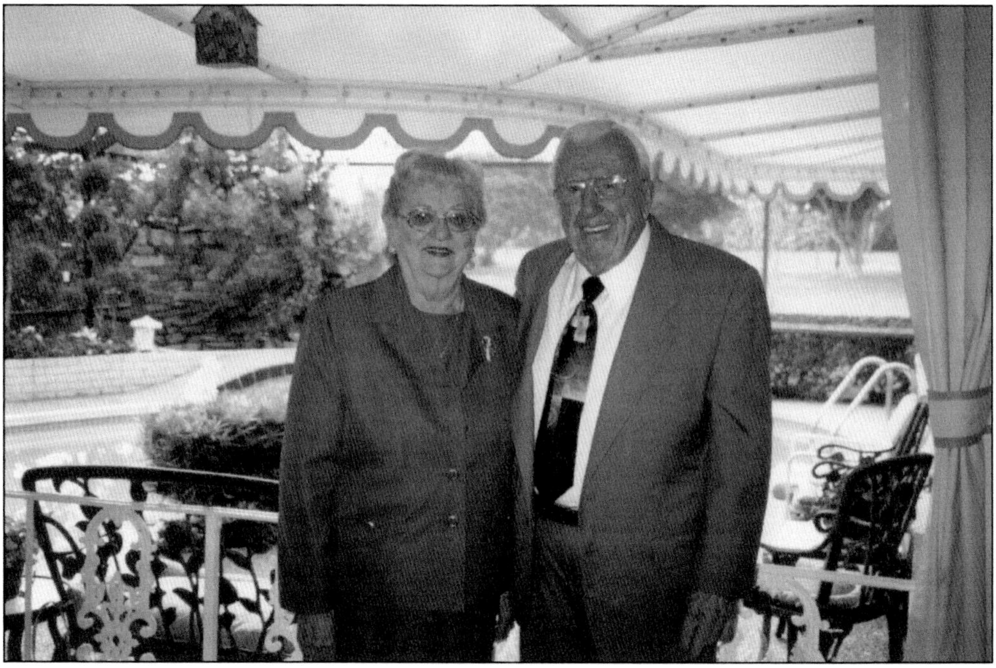

The LaChance Maternity Center was completed in 2001 and named for Leo and Theresa LaChance. Leo LaChance was a local realtor and land developer who was very involved with the hospital as a member of the board of trustees and a chairman of fundraising. The center revolutionized obstetrical care at Heywood Hospital. Birthing rooms allow patients to labor, deliver, and recover in the same bed. Ample space is provided for family members and equipment for the newborn's care. The 1921 West Wing delivery room was 172 square feet—small in comparison to today's birthing rooms with 425 square feet. In the image above are Leo and Theresa LaChance in Boca Raton, Florida. Below is a photograph of a birthing room. (Above, courtesy of Theresa LaChance.)

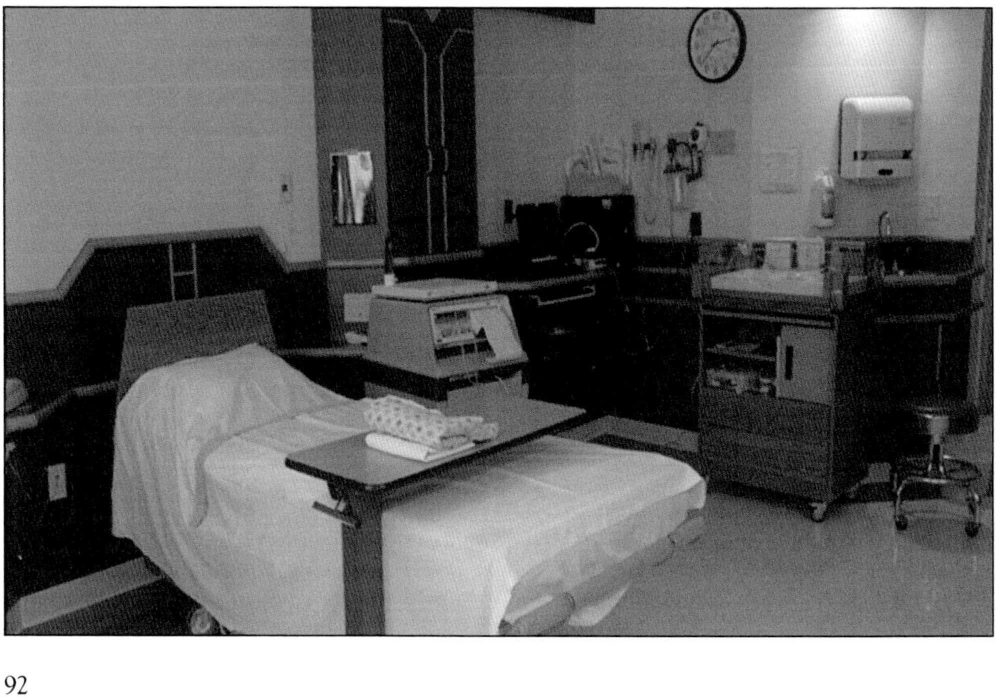

Postpartum rooms are single rooms allowing "rooming-in" as a comfortable option. More importantly, a fully equipped Cesarean-section room is located directly across the hall from the birthing rooms. In the former maternity ward, one had to navigate four double swinging doors, hallways, and an elevator to arrive at the operating room in the Favor Wing. Shown at right is the Cesarean-section operating room. Obstetrical patients especially appreciate a birthing tub, postpartum massage, breast feeding education, and a celebratory meal for the proud parents. A nursery for healthy newborns and another for those critically ill completes the LaChance Maternity Center. Shown below is the main nursery with a couple observing an infant through the window.

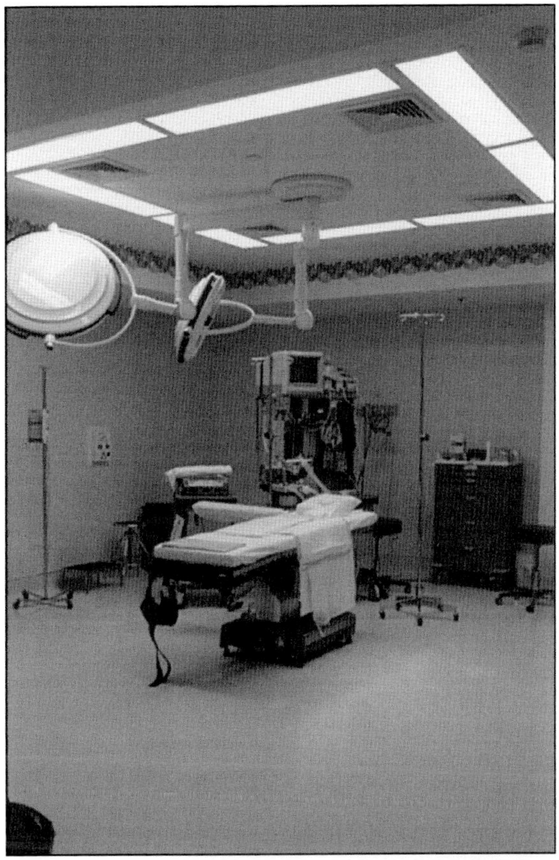

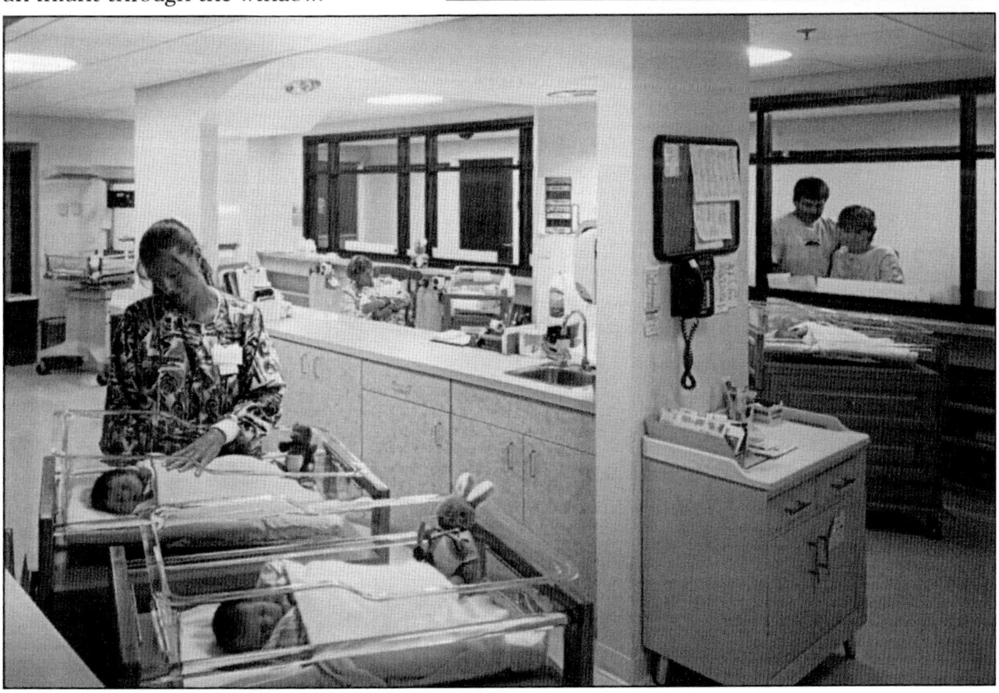

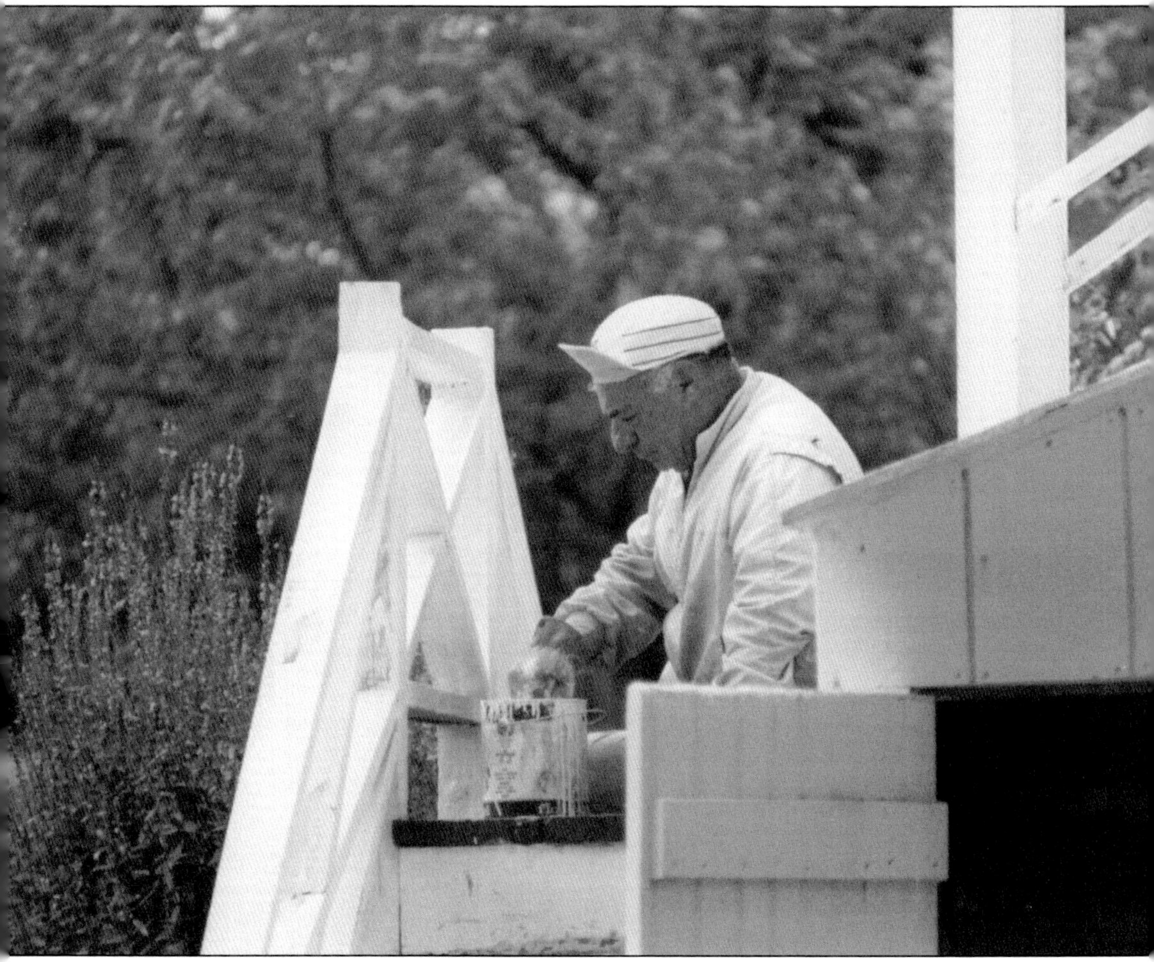

The pediatric department was moved in the mid-1990s from the West Wing to a smaller unit on the second floor of the Favor Wing. The move was made possible by the development of oral electrolyte solutions, such as Pedialyte, which allowed children suffering from an intestinal flu to be treated successfully as an outpatient. Also, new antibiotics and the ability to treat individuals with respiratory infections as outpatients reduced pediatric admissions. The new smaller unit was named for Dr. Rocco Raduazo, the first pediatrician to join Heywood Hospital. Raduazo was a practicing pediatrician at Heywood Hospital for many years. He gave his time and skills to the youth of Gardner as the local school and football team physician. He was loved by all, and a portrait of him still hangs in the pediatric unit today. In this image, Raduazo is putting a coat of paint on his home, which also served as his office for many years. (Courtesy of Sally Johnson.)

Eight

Volunteers through the Years

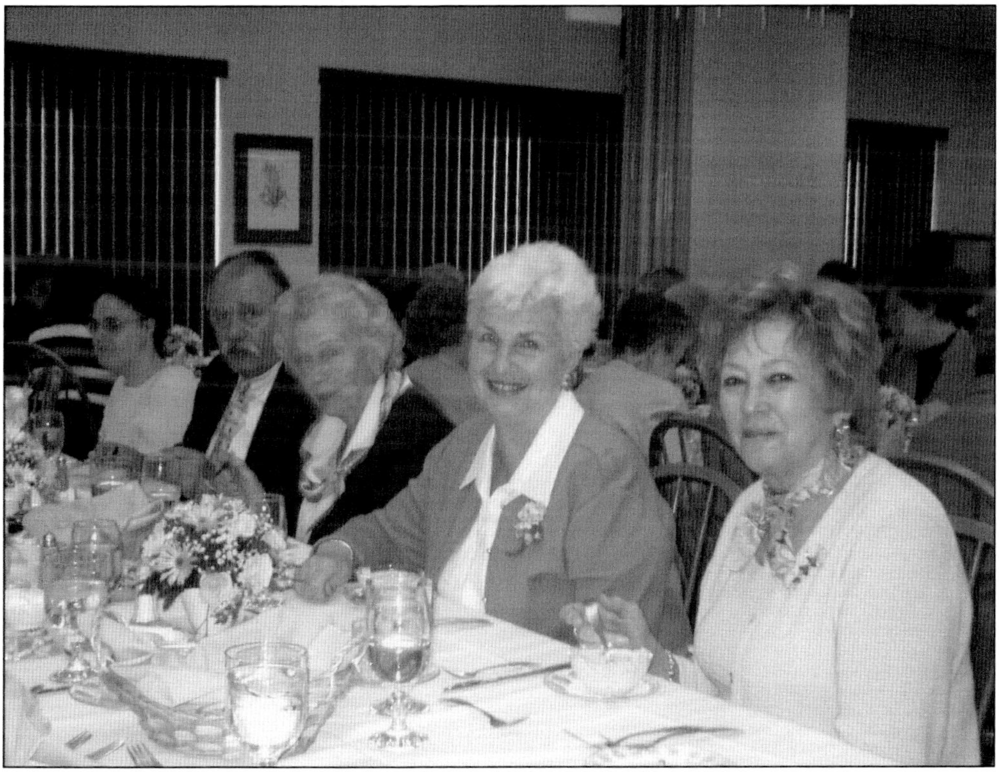

National Volunteer Week is celebrated throughout the country each April. Heywood Hospital honors its incredibly valuable volunteer force with an annual special appreciation and recognition dinner. It is an opportunity to thank the over 250 dedicated individuals who donate their time and talent to the institution as part of the hospital's volunteer program. Sue Deacon has been managing the volunteer program at Heywood Hospital since 1997

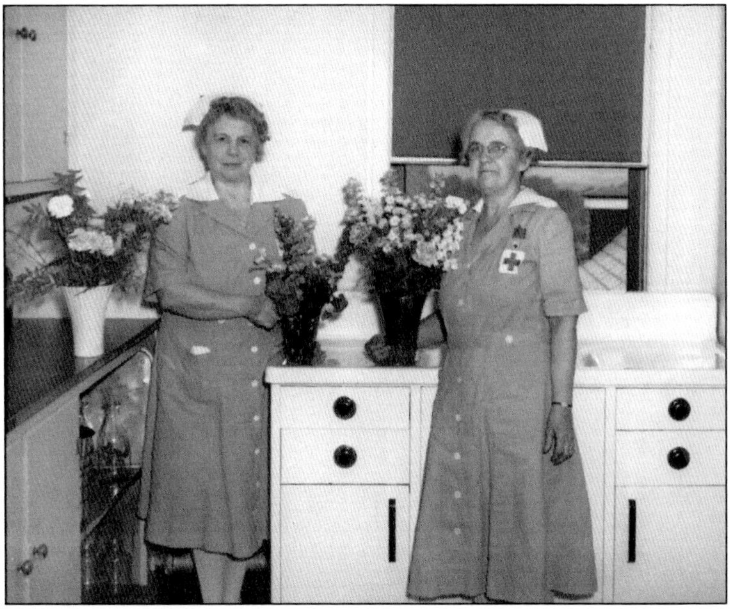

Mrs. Hill and Mrs. Snyder, pictured in 1947, were two members of a group of volunteers known as the Gray Ladies. The Gray Lady Service was part of the American Red Cross. The service began in 1918 at Walter Reed Army Hospital and spread to hospitals around the country. Dubbed the Gray Ladies because of the gray uniforms they wore, these volunteers provided nonmedical services to patients.

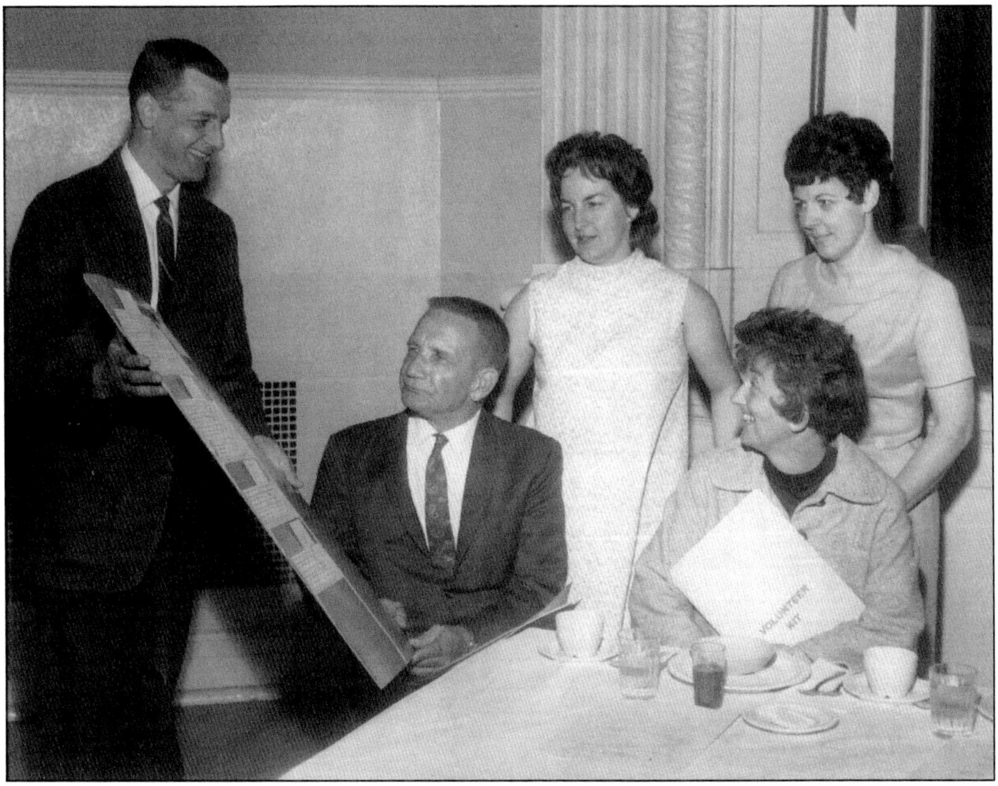

Today's adult volunteers in the volunteer program at Heywood Hospital are called senior volunteers and account for the bulk of the volunteers in the program. There is also a summer program for junior volunteers. The total hours worked by these volunteers averages over 42,000 annually, which equates to approximately $1 million in value. In this image, a group of new volunteers are being oriented.

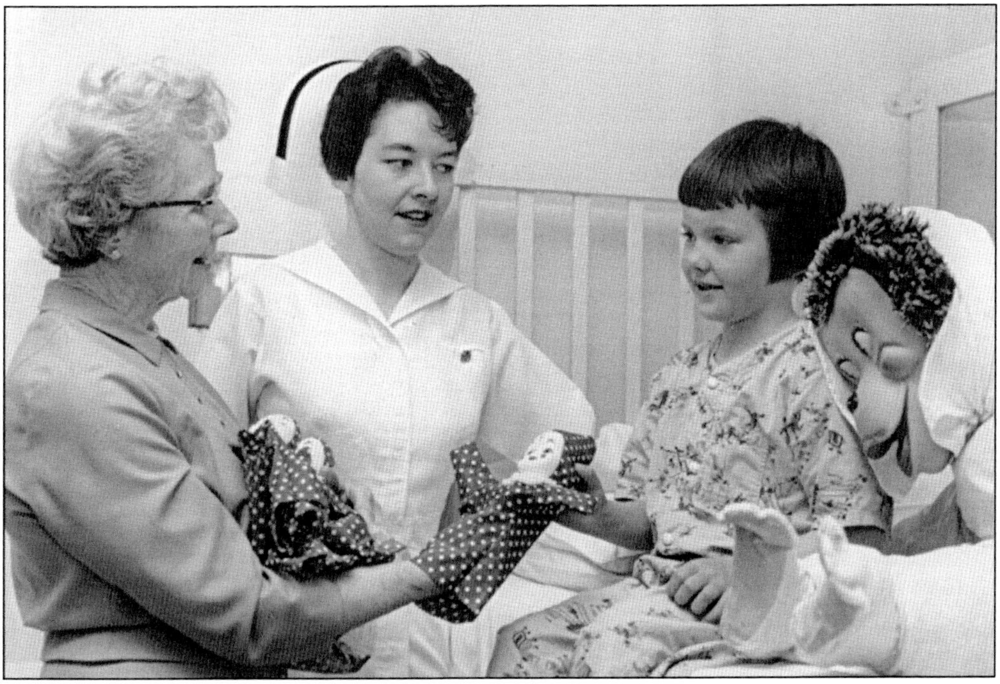

Crafting and distributing puppets to the children on the pediatric floor was a popular activity among volunteers. A total of 600 puppets were made one year. Many volunteers made the puppets, including church and scouting groups. This image shows a volunteer demonstrating how to make the puppet's head and arms move to a young patient who seems spellbound, as registered nurse Patricia Smith observes.

Martha Gearan (left) was the first director of the volunteer program in 1964 and founded the candy striper program at Heywood Hospital. Candy stripers were high school girls aged 14 to 18 who were given an opportunity to gain experience and learn skills in the medical field. Most were interested in being exposed to the nursing field.

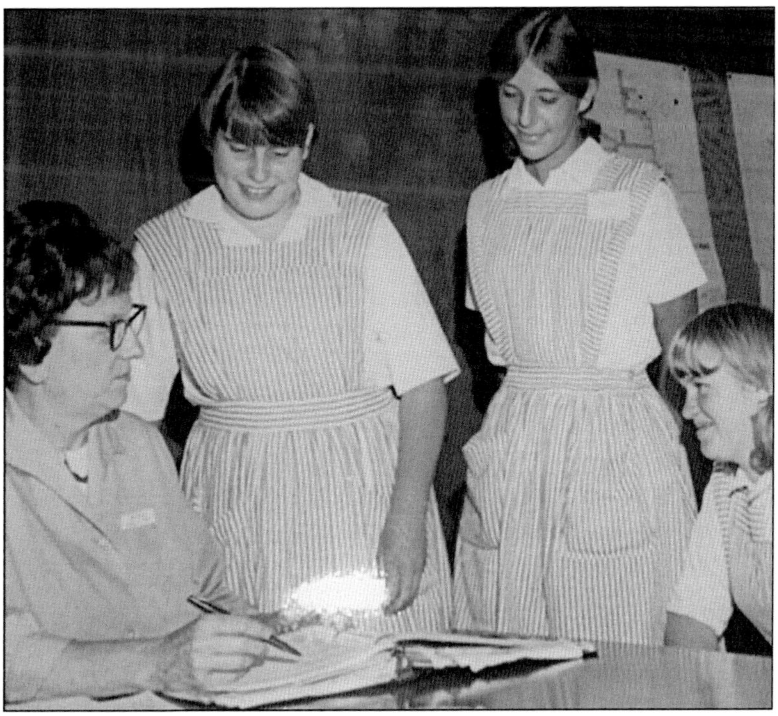

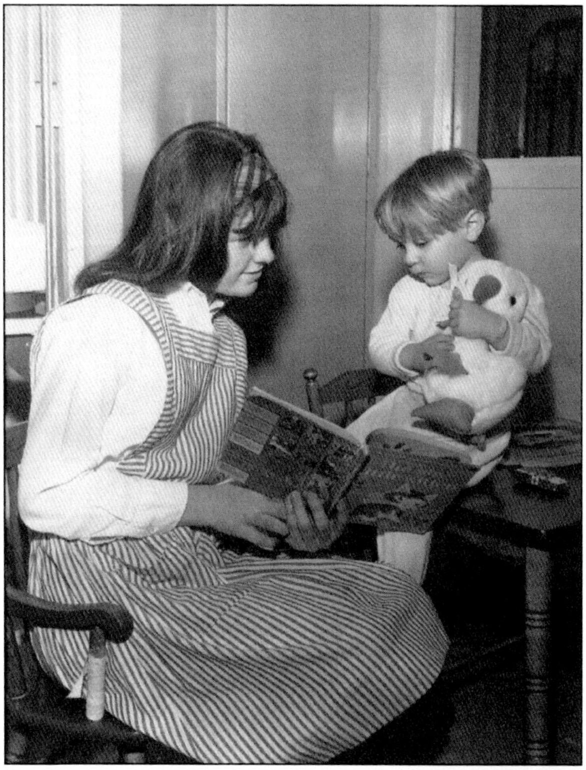

Some of the duties candy stripers performed for patients included refilling water pitchers, passing trays and refreshments, making unoccupied beds, assisting with stretcher and wheelchair transportation, and delivering flowers and newspapers. Today, the hospital has junior volunteers that include young men and women. Here, a candy striper reads to a pediatric patient.

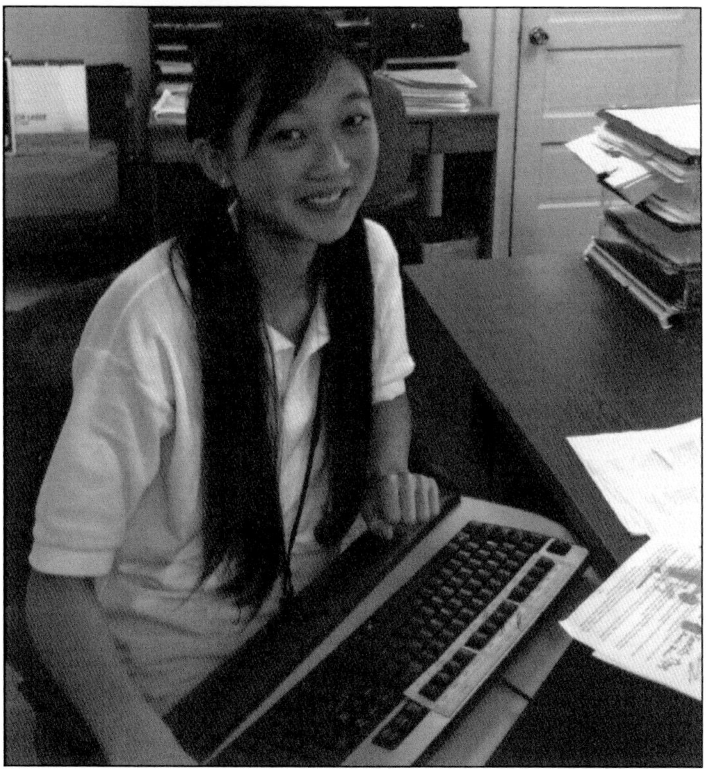

An outstanding junior volunteer is Emma Wang. Somehow, amidst attending camp at Massachusetts Institute of Technology's Center for Ultracold Atoms, earning her Gold Award from the Girl Scouts of America, and performing her duties as president of the Oakmont Environmental Association, Wang managed to find time to donate to the hospital, intending to continue her volunteer work in the future.

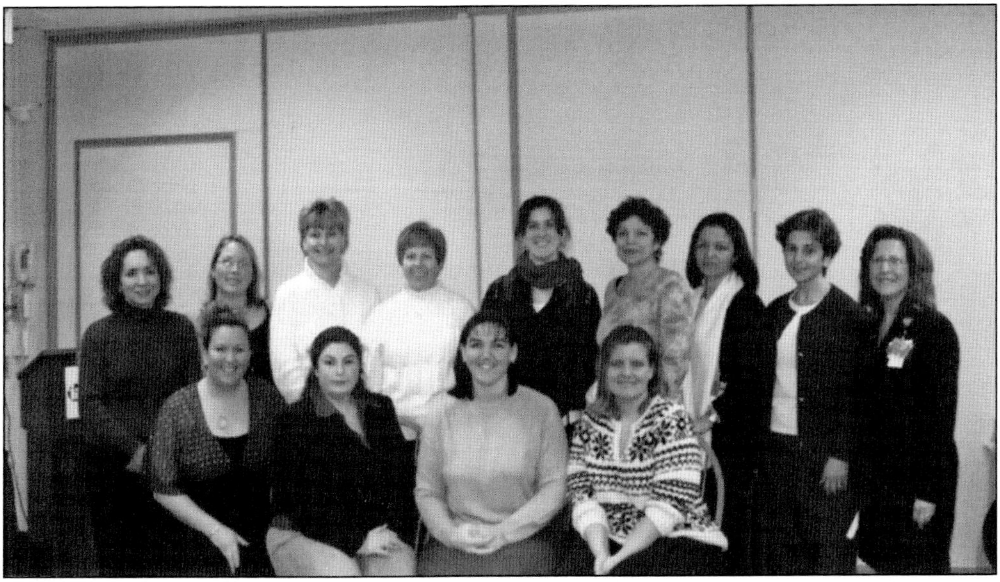

Doulas are a group of volunteers who are trained by the obstetrical unit to attend to the needs of labor patients and their families. They must commit to staying with the laboring patient until delivery. Last year, doulas donated over 10,000 hours of service. Seen here are volunteers from Heywood Hospital's doula program.

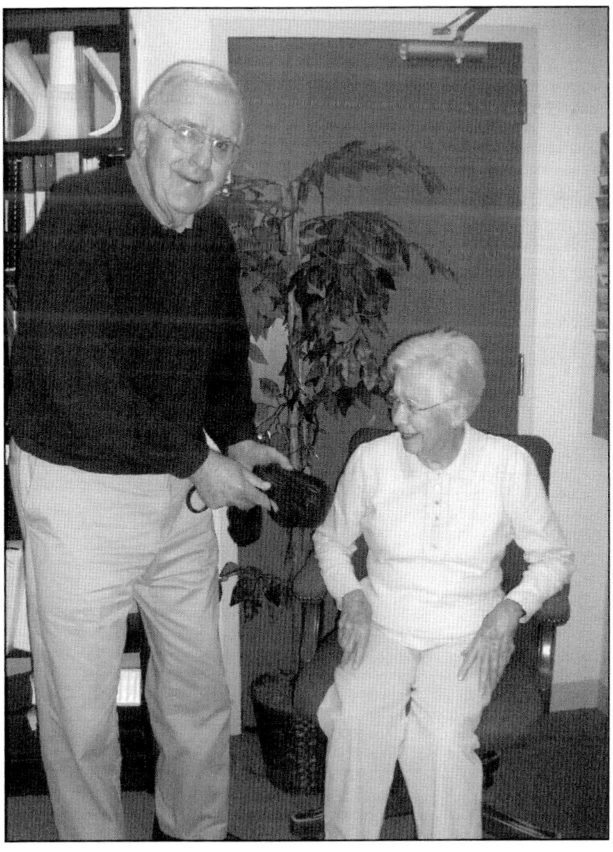

A major challenge for the elderly and others is to feel that they can reach medical help when alone and disabled. The answer is Lifeline. With this device, one only needs to push a button attached to the patient's clothing to receive assistance. In this image, volunteer Ed Stromski installs a Lifeline system for a patient in her home, which will allow her to continue living independently.

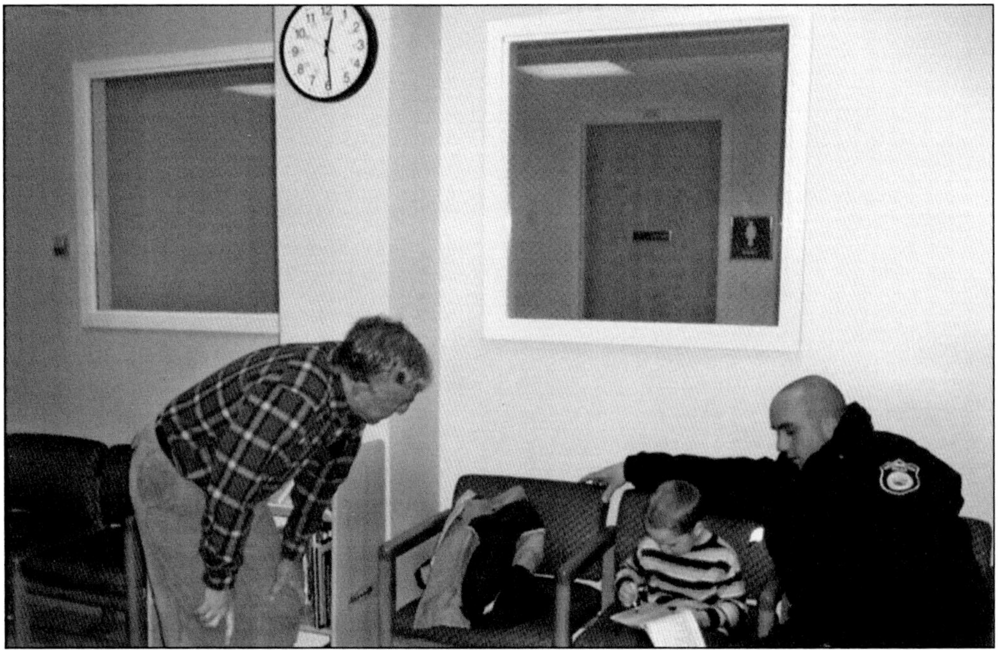

Emergency rooms are often very busy, resulting in prolonged waiting times. A key to a successful experience is for the patient to be informed regularly of what is transpiring in the emergency room and when one might expect to be seen. Retired pediatrician Dr. Donald Miller (left) volunteers assisting patients in the emergency room waiting area.

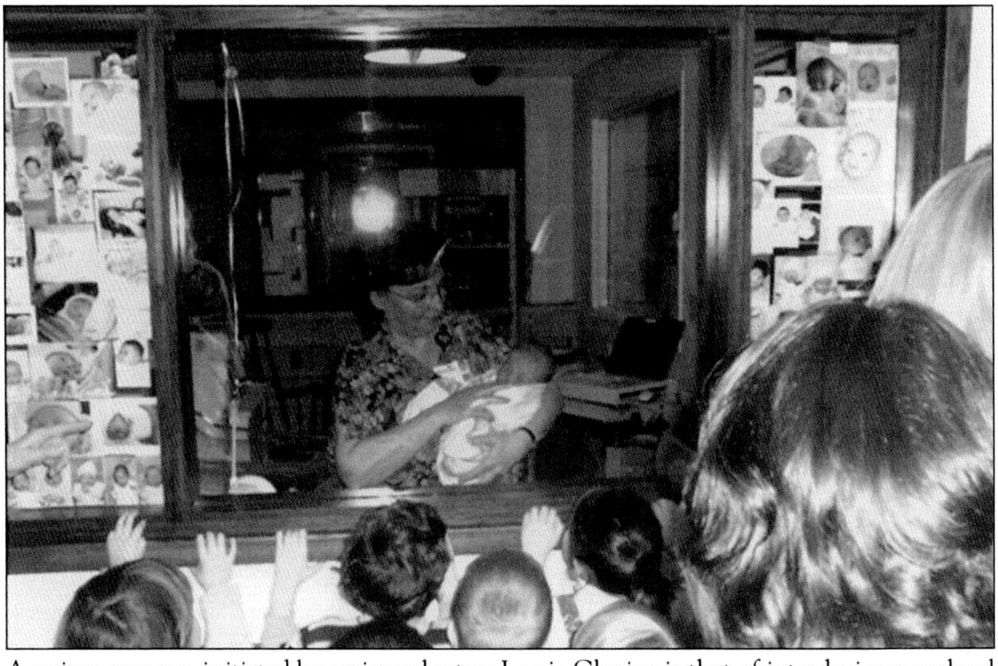

A unique program initiated by senior volunteer Lorrie Glovins is that of introducing preschool children to the hospital. The children are taken to the emergency room, radiology department, and the nursery. They love to view X-rays. Seen here with their parents, the preschool children are enthralled by the newborns in the nursery.

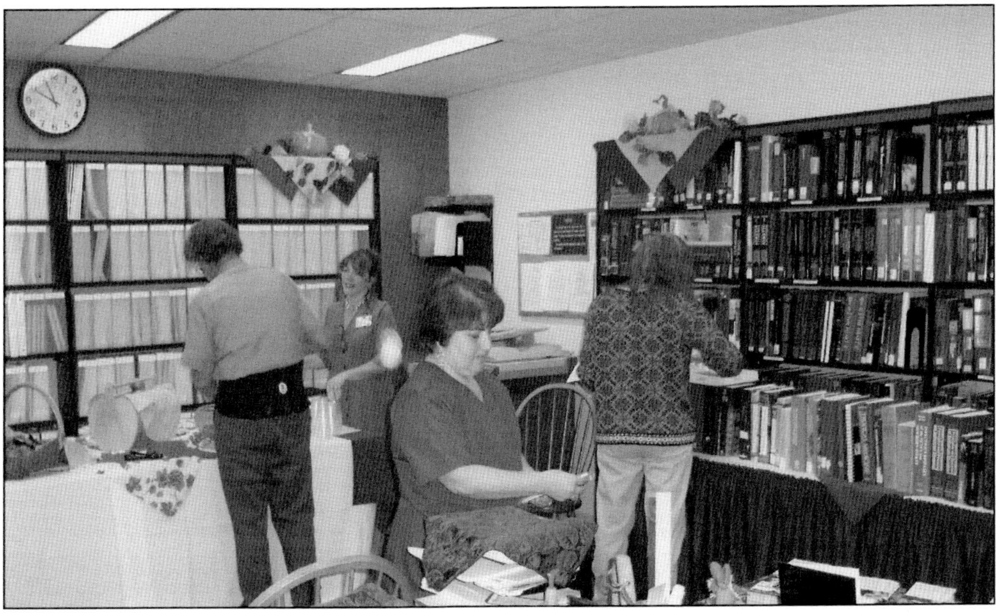

The Heywood Hospital Health Sciences Library, located next to the cafeteria, serves the entire hospital community, including physicians, nurses, hospital staff, patients, and community residents. Joan Blast volunteers her time in both the gift shop and the hospital library. For over 11 years, she has assisted in providing information resources to the library's patrons. On her 80th birthday, Blast skydived—free falling from 13,500 feet—at Jumptown in Orange, Massachusetts, the first commercial skydiving center in the United States. She is contemplating a second jump to celebrate her 85th birthday. Looking proud as punch after her jump, Blast is the embodiment of the can-do spirit of Heywood Hospital's volunteers. (Both, courtesy of Joan Blast.)

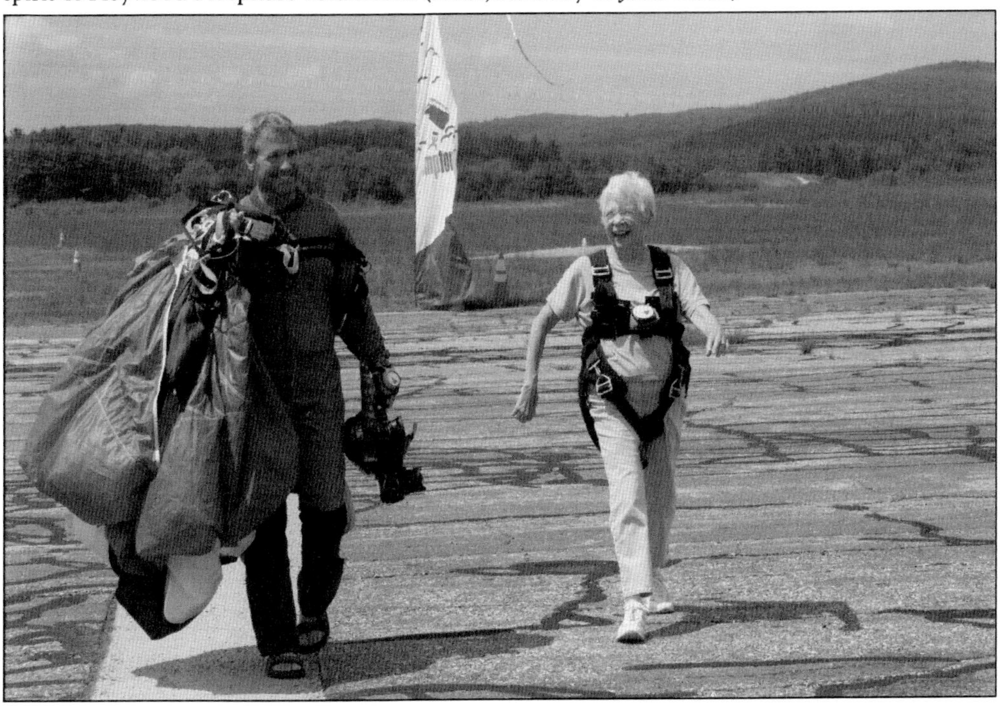

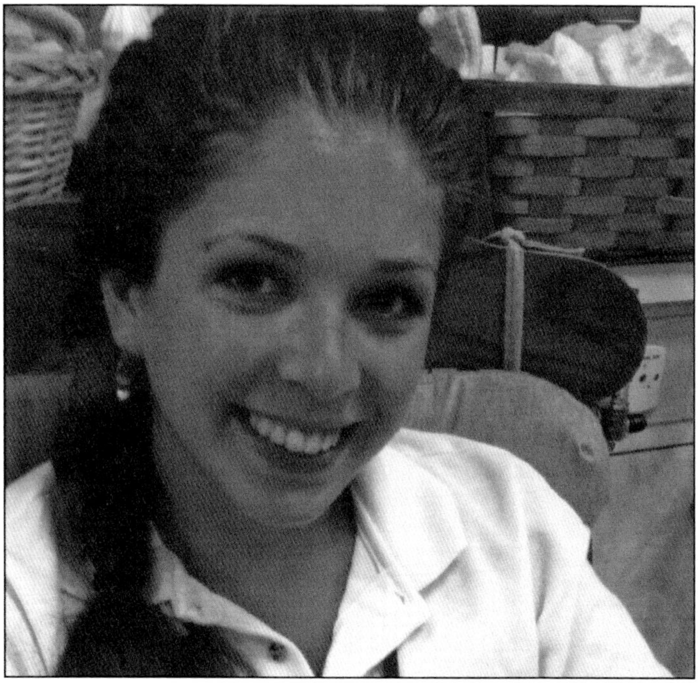

Volunteers are extremely important to Heywood Hospital. Likewise, Heywood Hospital provides very important educational opportunities and satisfying experiences for volunteers. Junior volunteer Jennifer Antocci shares her thoughts: "My experience on this floor [obstetrics] was so profound that it gave me the basis for my college essay. Community service is a wonderful thing, and giving your time to an institution such as Heywood Hospital is a warming and humbling experience."

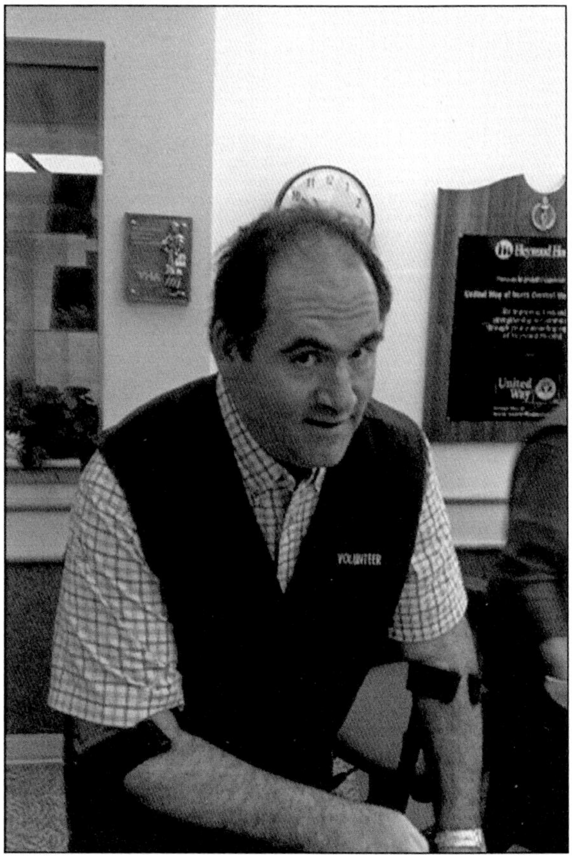

This heartfelt testimonial is from senior volunteer David Savoie: "Being a volunteer with Heywood Hospital has truly enriched my life. As volunteers, we give of ourselves, but we receive much more—self-respect, pride in a job well done, and the joy in meeting and assisting wonderful people. Thank you so much, Heywood Hospital, for accepting me as part of your volunteer program." Thank *you*, David! Thanks to *all*!

Nine

Fundraisers and Festivities

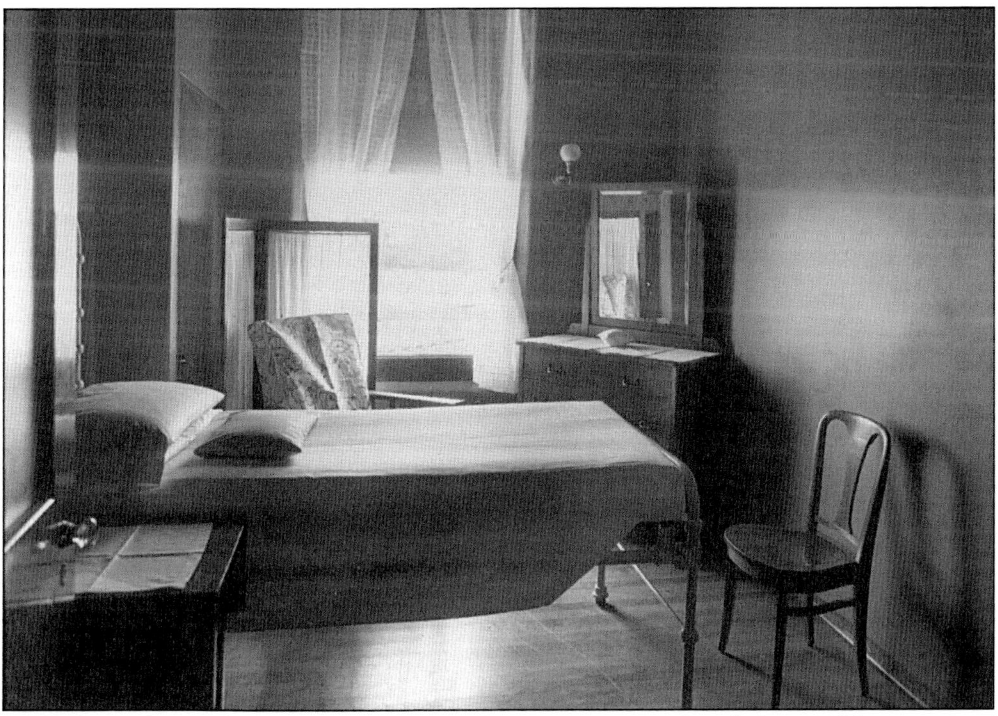

The Henry Heywood Memorial Hospital Aid Association was founded in 1927 by a group of women who felt they had something to contribute to the hospital, and they certainly did. Initially, they raised money via card games and dues. The first year, they raised $1,061.36 for linens for the hospital, as seen here.

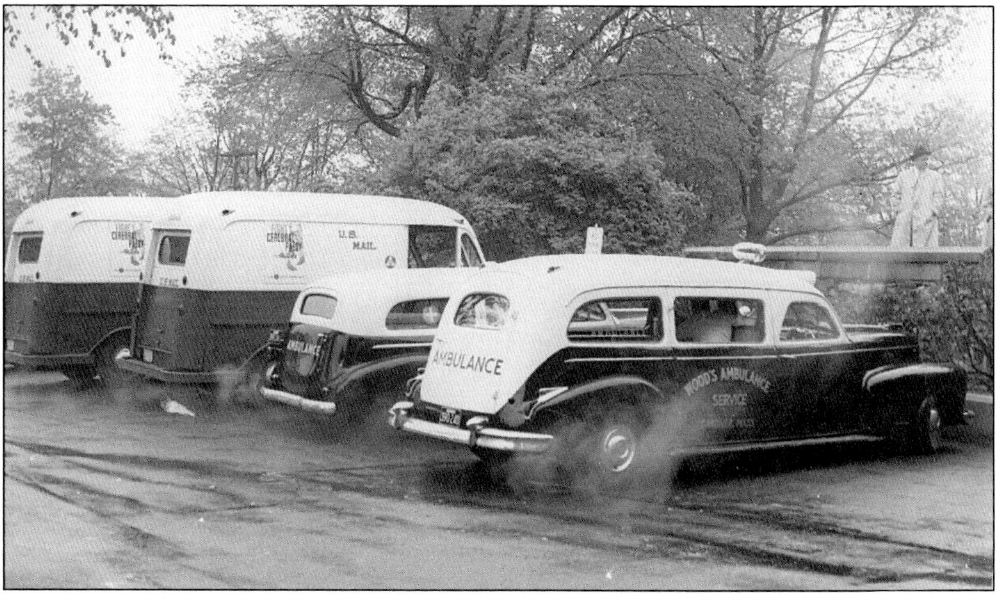

Street fairs were popular fundraisers from 1937 through 1944. The town would close the portion of Cross Street between Elm and Lawrence Streets. In 1970, a fair held on Waterford Street was called the Red Stocking Fair. Red stockings were sold, attached to automobile antennas, and driven about town. The Henry Heywood Memorial Hospital Aid Association's first large purchase was a 1942 Chevrolet ambulance costing $3,250 (second vehicle from right)

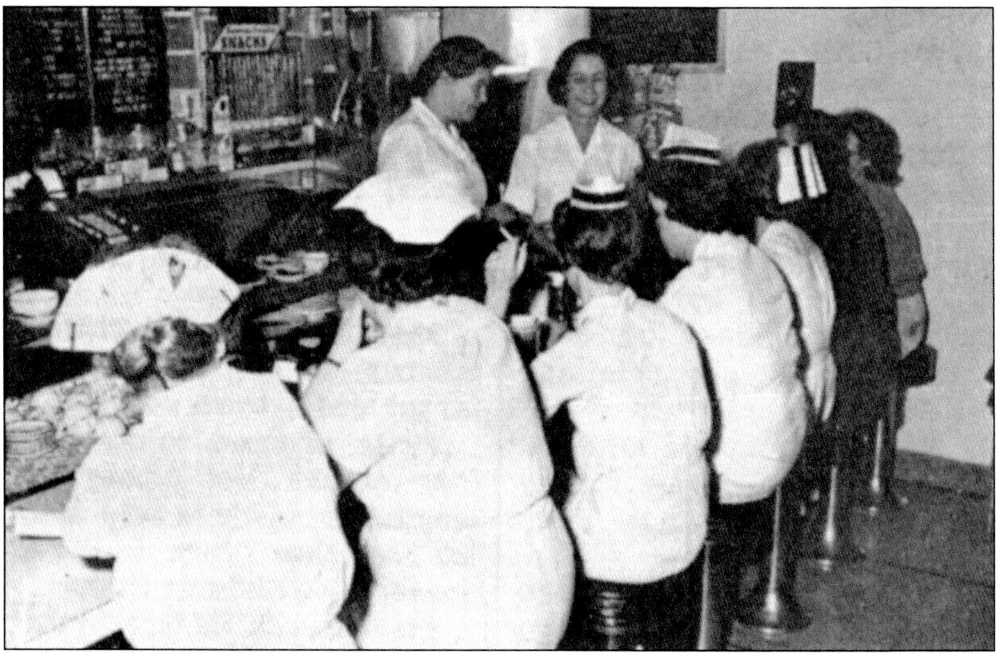

A snack bar was opened in the West Wing in 1955. The Henry Heywood Memorial Hospital Aid Association financed the project with a $3,500 loan that the hospital repaid within three years. With nine stools and three tables, it was a popular spot for staff during coffee break. There was a paid manager as well as volunteer workers. Volunteers baked pies and cakes to be sold to customers.

In spite of a new bar and furniture of modern design as shown here, the snack bar was closed in 1983. High taxes, the need for more salaried help, and the new hospital cafeteria that provided similar food and snacks all played a role in the closing of what was once a highly lucrative project for what became known as the Hospital Aid Association (HAA).

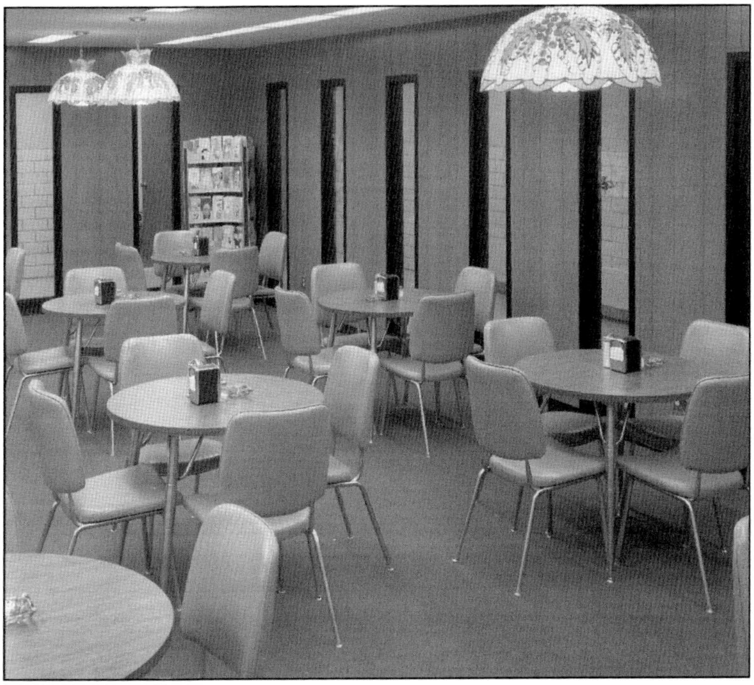

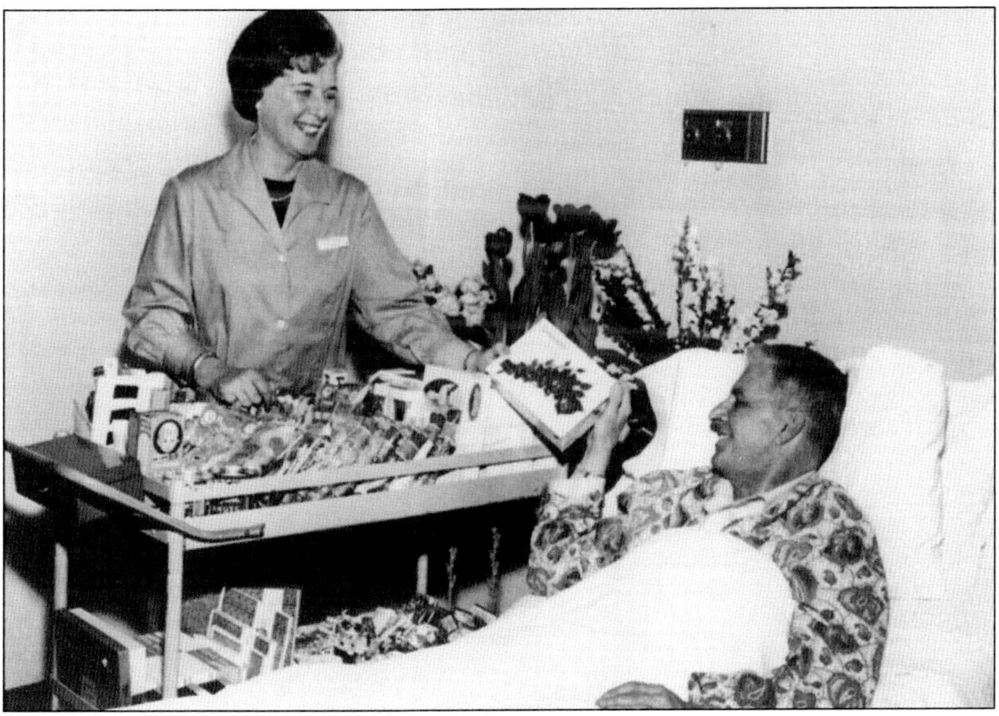

A gift cart called the "Pink Cadillac" was initiated in 1963. A volunteer pushed the cart through the hospital corridors three times per week. Patients could purchase toiletries and other necessary items. Here, HAA volunteer Geri Knitzer sells a box of candy to Volney Howe, member of the board of trustees and descendent of early settlers of Gardner. A conference room at the hospital was named for Howe.

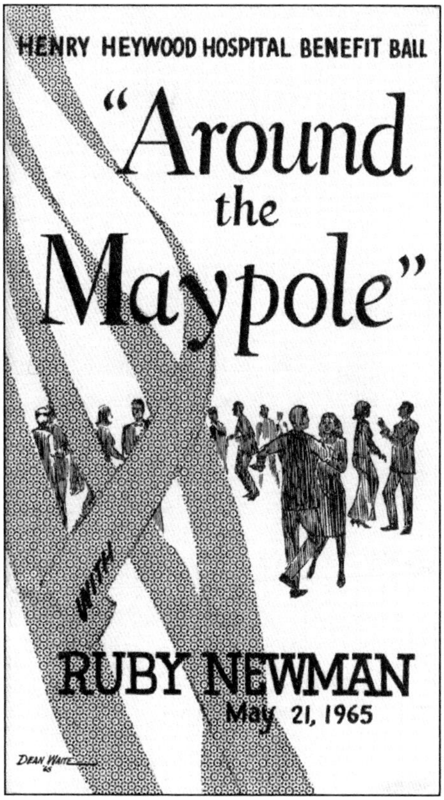
HENRY HEYWOOD HOSPITAL BENEFIT BALL
"Around the Maypole"
WITH
RUBY NEWMAN
May 21, 1965

Annual benefit balls were popular fundraisers from 1959 to 1979. Dances were semiformal and held locally at the National Guard Armory. Well-known bands were invited and included Ralph Flanagan, Ray Moulton and his orchestra, and Ruby Newman. As alcoholic beverages were not served in the armory, plenty of "tailgating" occurred in the parking lot. The Around the Maypole benefit ball was held in 1965.

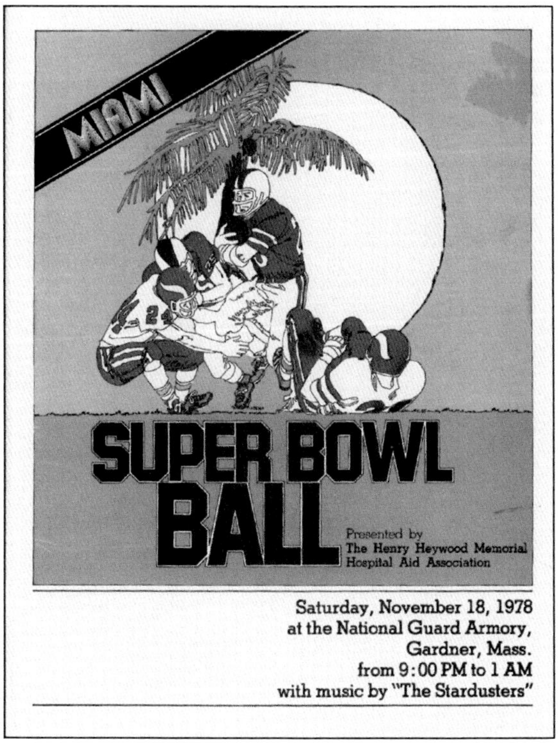

The benefit balls required considerable planning and work by the HAA members. The hall was elaborately decorated. Tickets and advertising in the brochure had to be sold. Year after year, the HAA came up with imaginative themes and ideas for fundraising. This is the brochure cover for the popular Super Bowl Ball held at the armory in 1978.

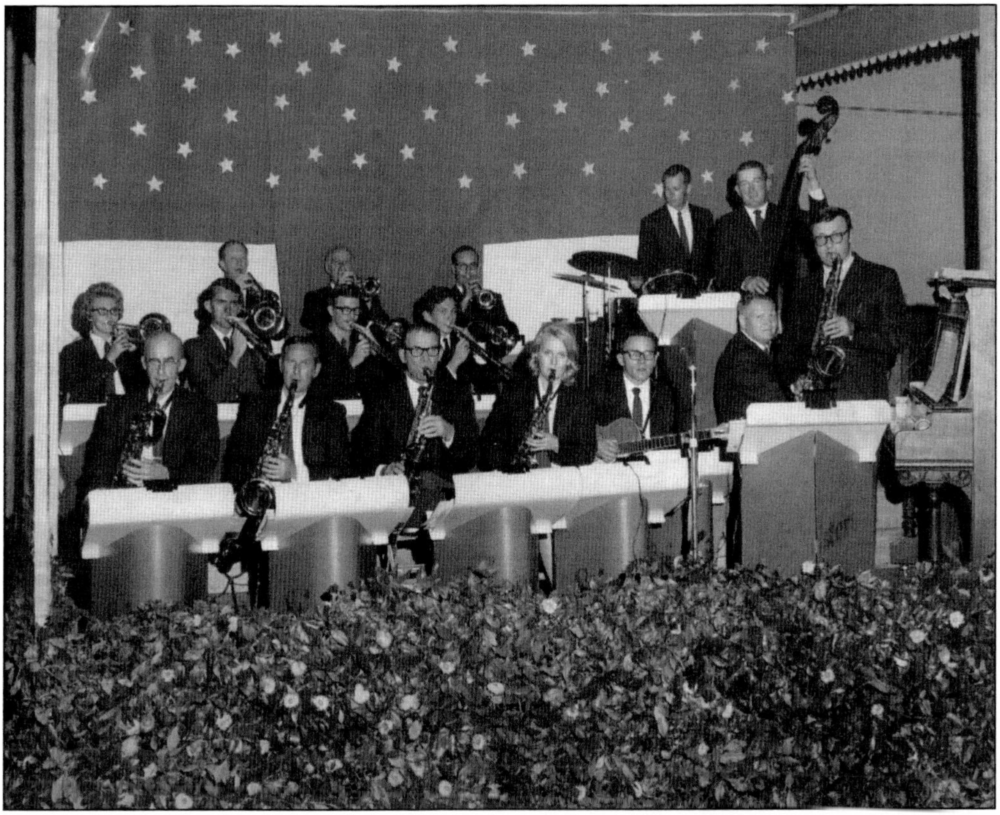

The Stardusters were a local band led by Mel Ostroff, of the Standard Chair Furniture Company in Gardner. They performed at the 1969 and 1971 benefit balls and at concerts in 1986 and 1987 for the HAA. Ostroff (far right) is pictured above playing the saxophone for a benefit at the armory in November 1969. *High Fever Follies* was presented in 1966, 1967, and 1977. Real "talent" performed in front of a live audience in the Elm Street High School auditorium. *High Fever Follies* 1977 commemorated the 50th anniversary of the HAA. The performance was directed by New York City's Ric Sanford, who was paid to produce the show.

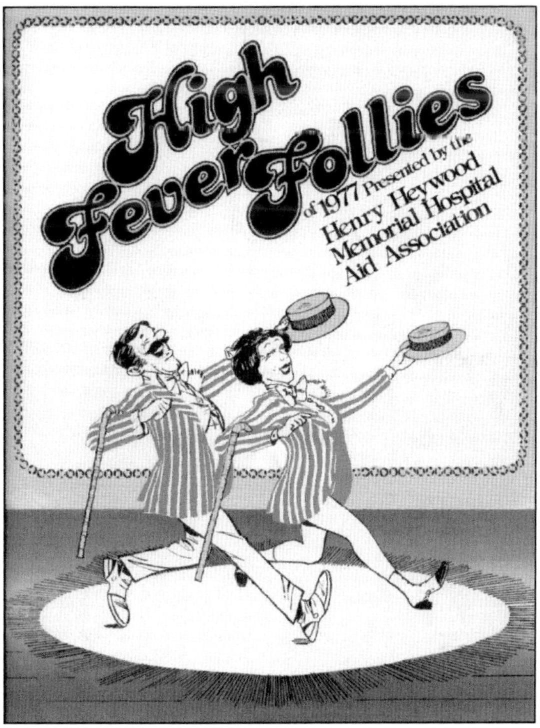
High Fever Follies
of 1977 Presented by the
Henry Heywood
Memorial Hospital
Aid Association

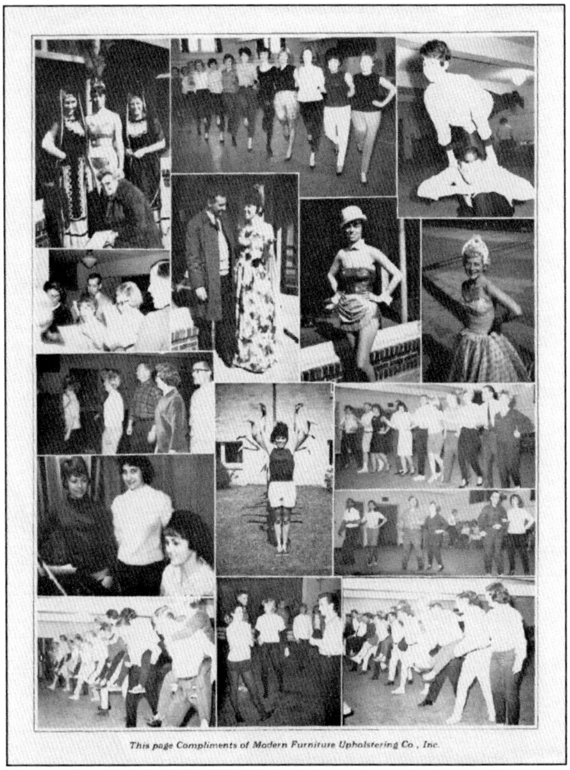

It was difficult to be sure who had more fun—the actors or the audience. This photograph shows a collage of images depicting performers practicing a variety of dances and skits. It adorned the 1967 *High Fever Follies* program. The master of ceremonies was Gardner dentist Dr. Charles Martel.

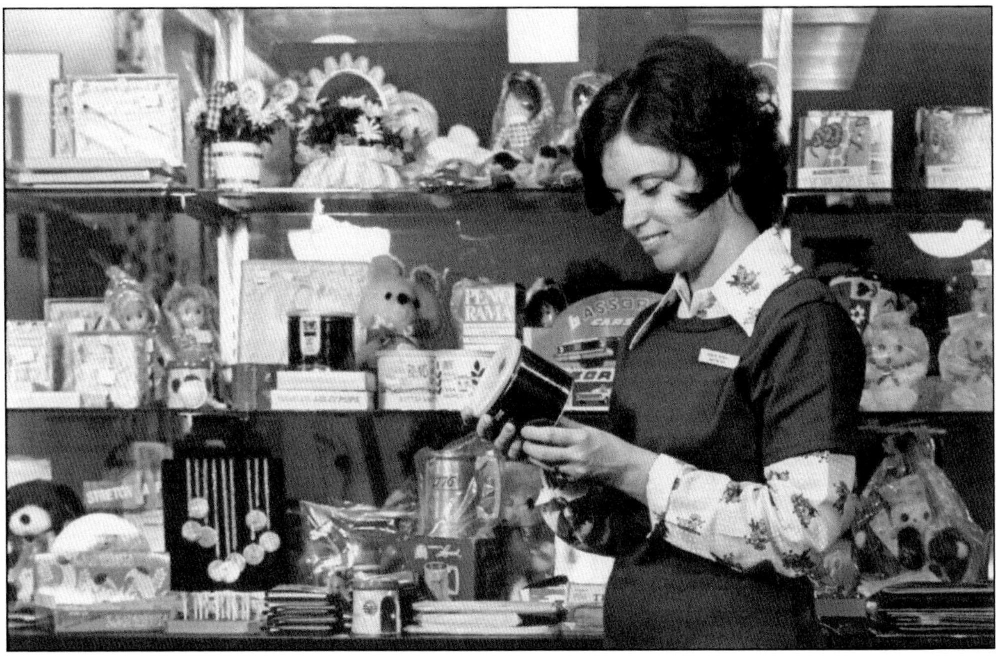

A gift shop was opened in 1970. Shortly thereafter, a separate area near the hospital entrance was dedicated to the gift shop. It is interesting that the best seller for the gift shop was the series of Beanie Babies. They were so popular that when a new order came in, the sale was limited to nighttime. Once, there was actually a skirmish over a position in line.

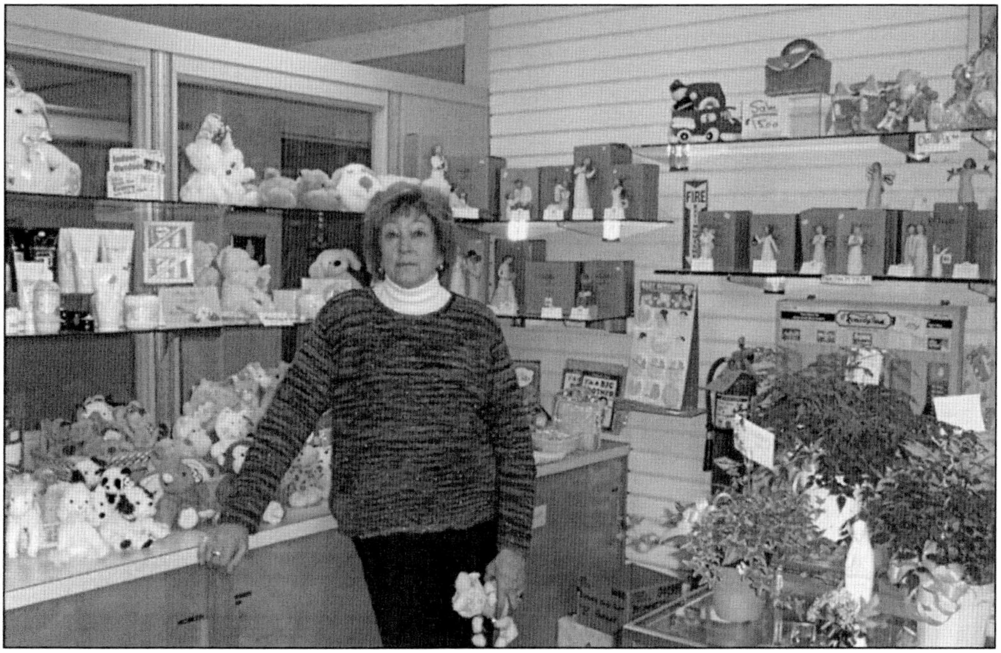

Most gift shops in hospitals are managed and financed by the hospital. However, Heywood Hospital's gift shop has always been managed and manned by volunteers. This image shows the many items on the shelves for children and adults. Pictured is Elaine Colombo, who voluntarily managed the gift shop for 25 years.

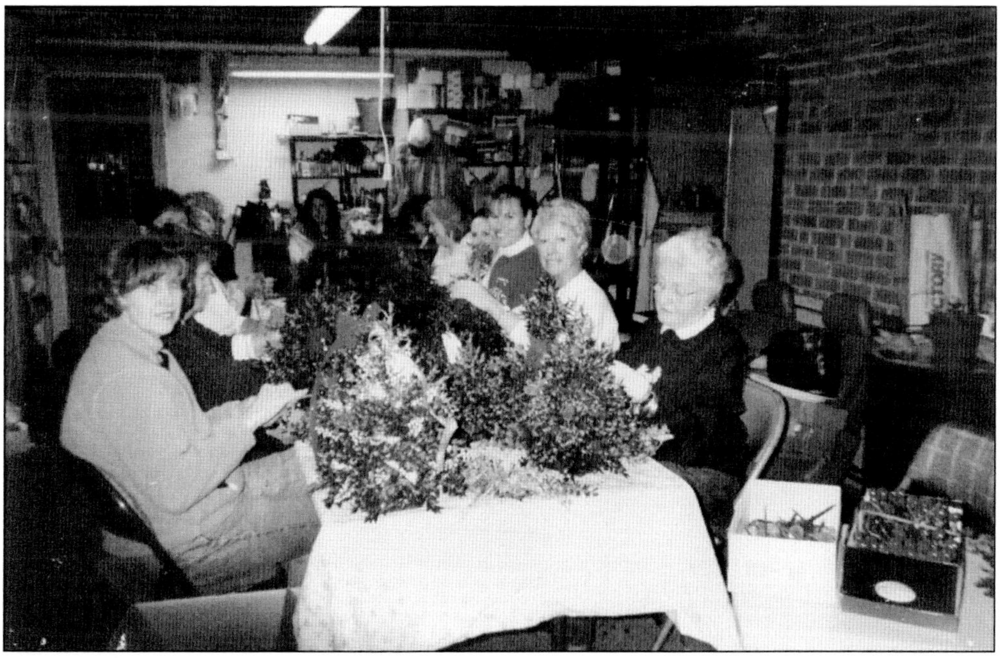

Since 1986, the Evergreen Fair has been a primary fundraiser for the HAA. It is held prior to Christmas, and HAA members make beautiful wreaths, swags, and boxwood trees. Homemade cakes, pies, and crafts are sold. Hospital departments and physicians' offices contribute large baskets with items of various themes for a Chinese auction. Here members craft boxwood trees.

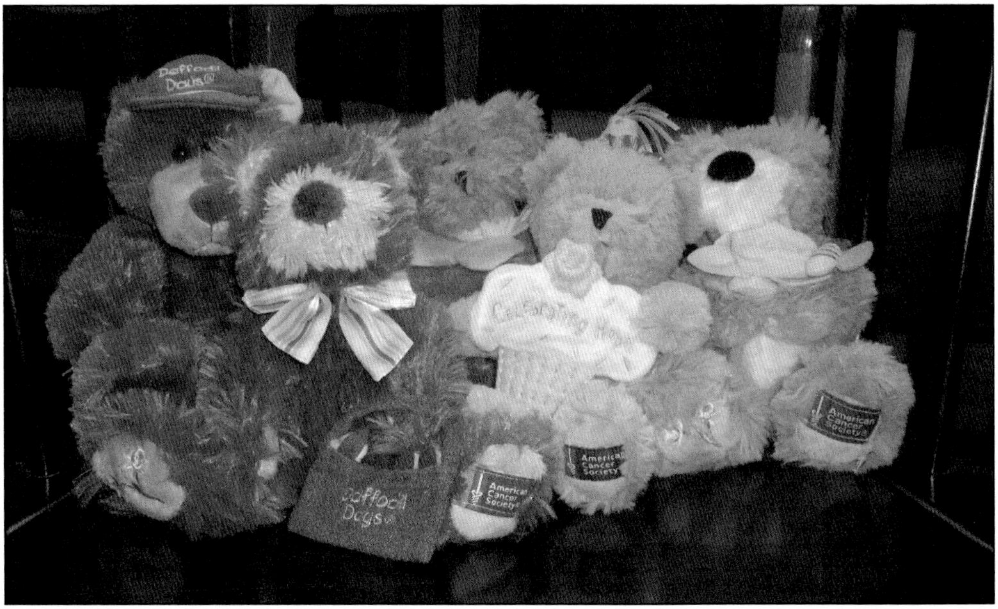
Daffodil Days
American Cancer Society

Daffodils have been an annual reminder to all of the great work done by the Hospital Aid Association. Each March, daffodils and teddy bears are sold to raise money for the American Cancer Society. They are also distributed to hospital inpatients. An early volunteer services manual rightly states, "A smiling happy volunteer is always a bouquet for the patient."

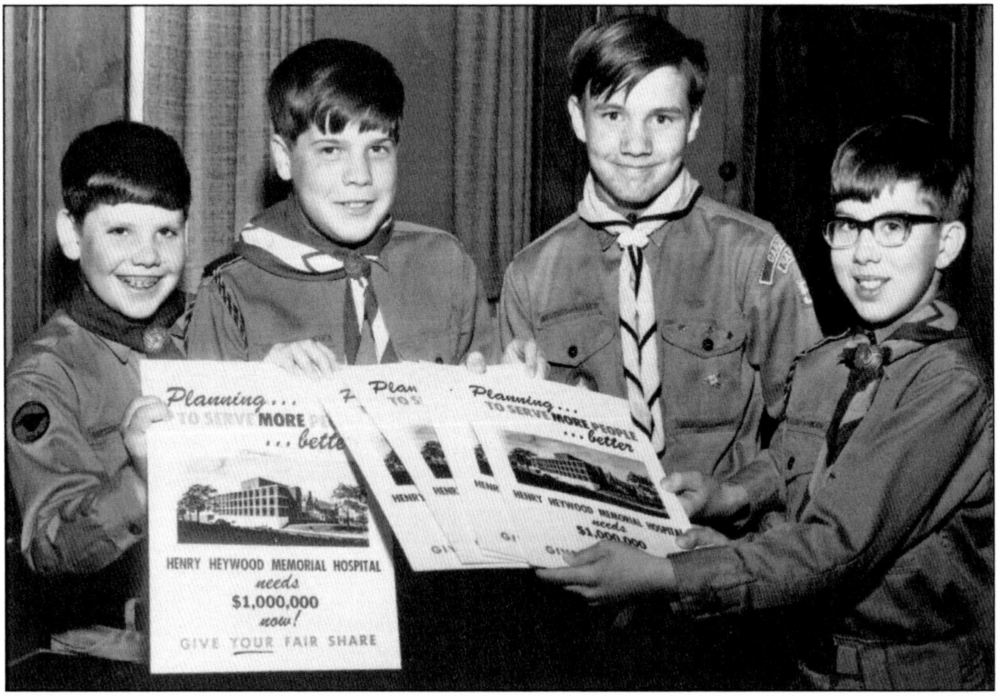
Planning...
TO SERVE MORE PEOPLE
... better
HENRY HEYWOOD MEMORIAL HOSPITAL
needs
$1,000,000
now!
GIVE YOUR FAIR SHARE

The community gives much back to the hospital in terms of monetary funds during capital campaigns. Most campaigns have coincided with major building projects. During the Expansion and Development Fund campaign of 1968, local Boy Scout troops did their part to help promote the fundraiser by distributing campaign posters to local businesses.

The 1959 capital campaign coincided with the construction of the Favor Wing and its first two floors, including the emergency room, surgical suite, and medical surgical ward. In this image of the groundbreaking ceremony for that project are, from left to right, Robert Keyworth Sr., chairman of the board Charles Brooks, Mayor Cyril Landry, and Dr. Leonard Thompson.

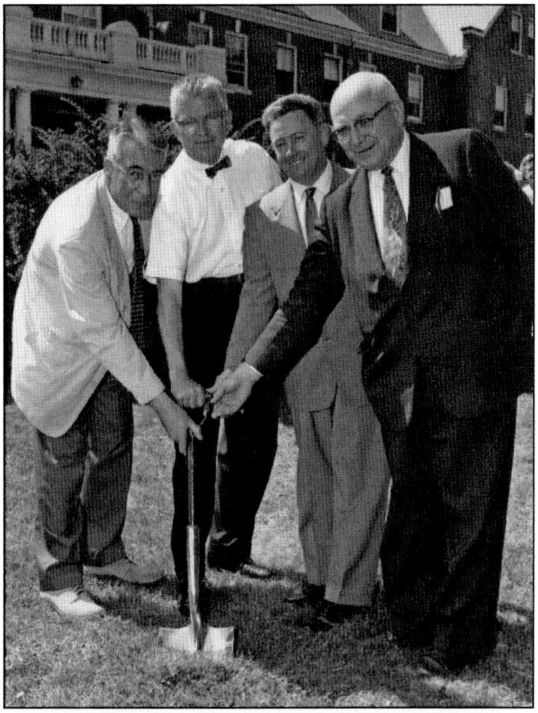

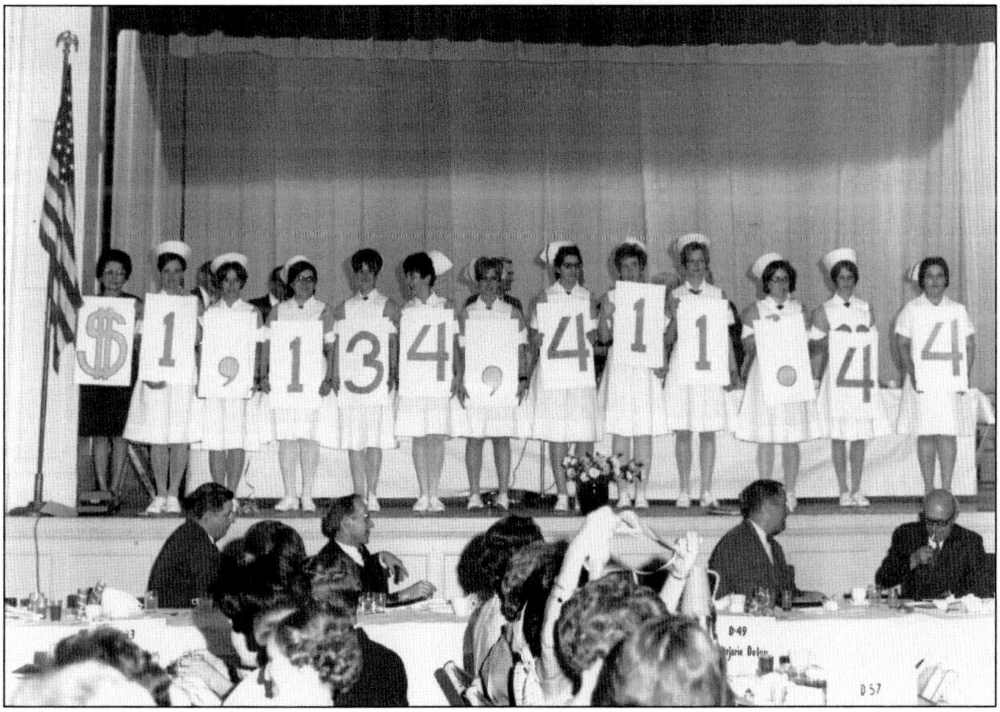

The 1968 Expansion and Development Fund campaign had a goal of $1 million. It surpassed its goal by more than $134,000. The theme was Planning to Serve More People Better. The money helped to fund the top two additional floors of the Favor Wing, the new kitchen and cafeteria, a new snack bar, and a combination physicians' library and conference room.

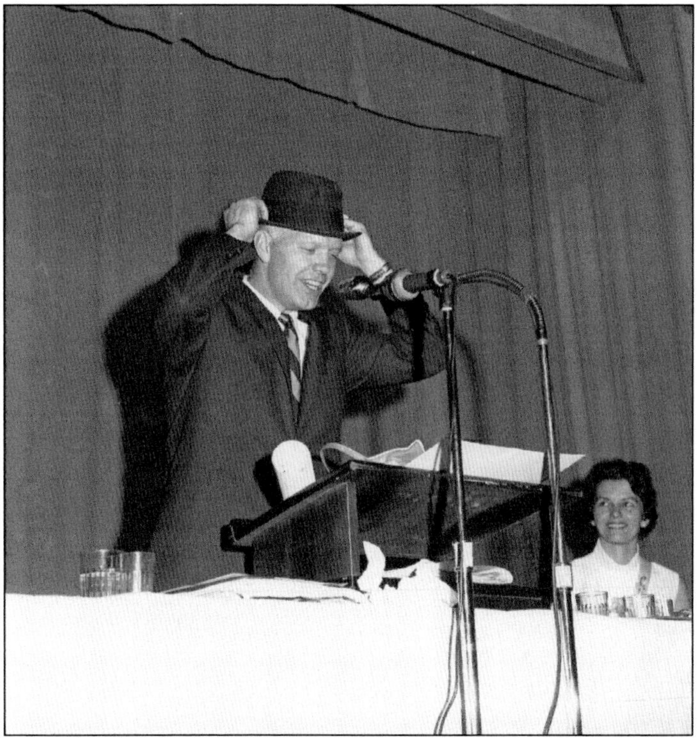

Harold "Jay" Drake presided over the 1968 campaign. Drake was a longtime friend of Heywood Hospital and served on the board of trustees for many years. Always good for a laugh, Drake awarded miniature airline travel bags in lieu of "trips to Europe" as gifts to campaign fundraisers and contributors at the victory dinner.

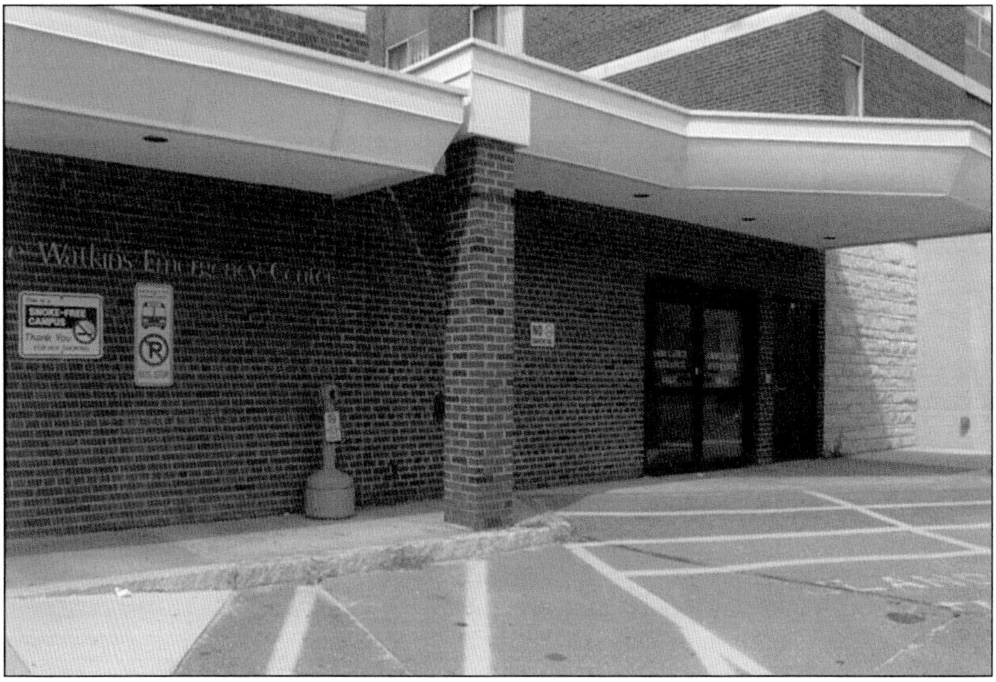

The Caring for the Future campaign of 1990 was cochaired by Leo LaChance and Thomas Kelly. Donations helped to fund the Watkins Emergency Center, pictured here. The New Century campaign in 1999 raised funds toward the LaChance Maternity Center, Thomas P. Kelly Ambulatory Care Center, and the Edward I. Stromski Oncology Center.

An important annual fundraiser is the Heywood Hospital Golf Classic. The first annual Golf Classic was held on June 21, 1993. The event was conceived when Tom Kelly, Jim Faust, and Chris Watkins met at the office of Simplex Time Recorder Company. Watkins proposed an annual golf tournament at Oak Hill Country Club for the friends of Heywood Hospital. This is the cover of the first banquet brochure.

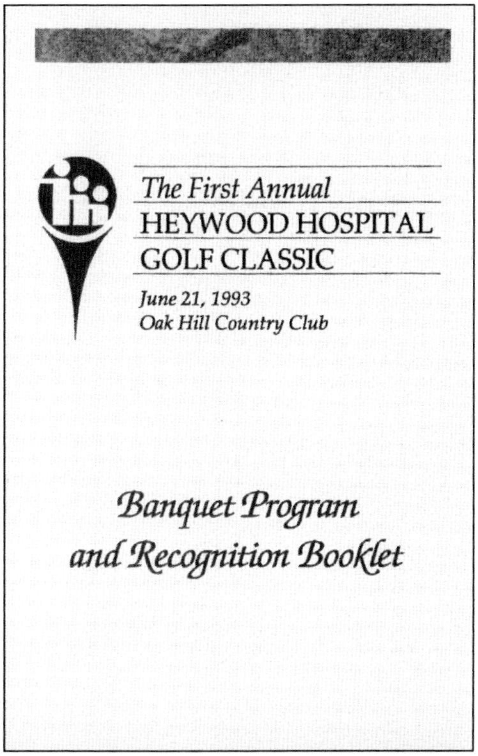

The First Annual
HEYWOOD HOSPITAL
GOLF CLASSIC

June 21, 1993
Oak Hill Country Club

Banquet Program
and Recognition Booklet

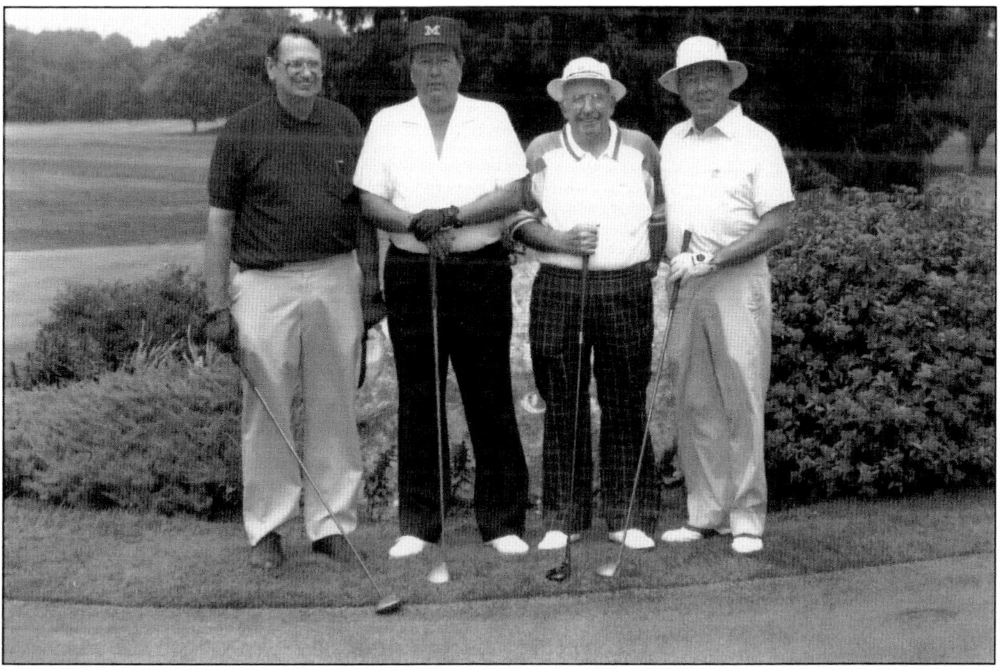

The event included lunch, a day of golf, an elegant cocktail party, and a dinner banquet. Profits have benefited many hospital entities such as capital equipment and building projects. Here is a photograph of the first foursome off the first tee at Oak Hill Country Club in 1993. From left to right are Jim Faust, Chris Watkins, Leo LaChance, and Tom Kelly.

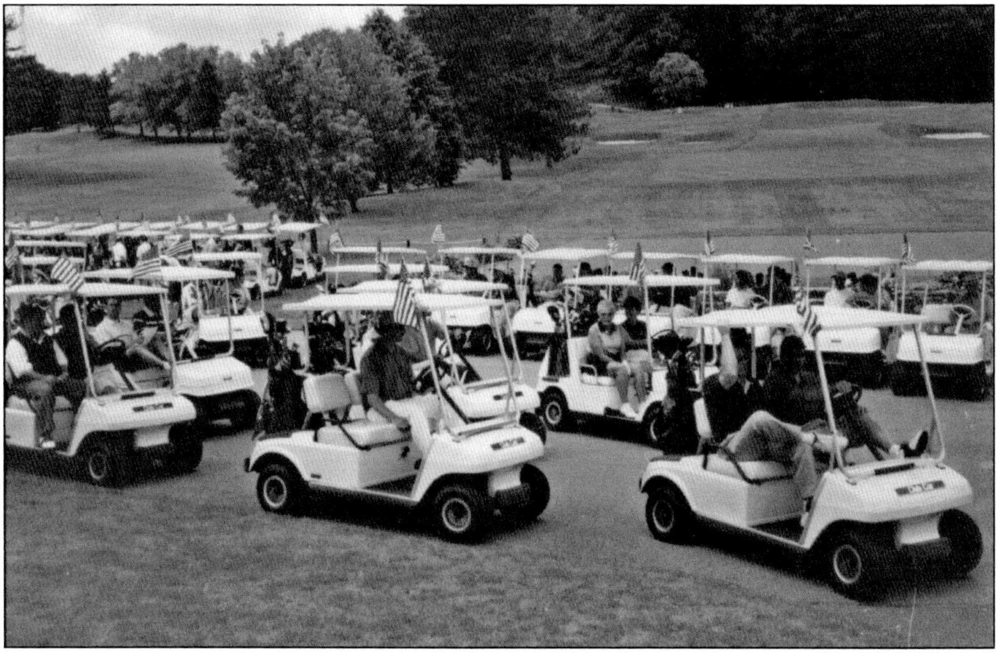

Much of the success of the Heywood Hospital Golf Classic is thanks to golf professional Jim O'Leary and the culinary skills of Oak Hill Country Club's chef. The taking-off of the carts for the appropriate tees is one of the great sights. Flags representing Heywood Hospital, the United States of America, and a cure for cancer adorn the golf carts.

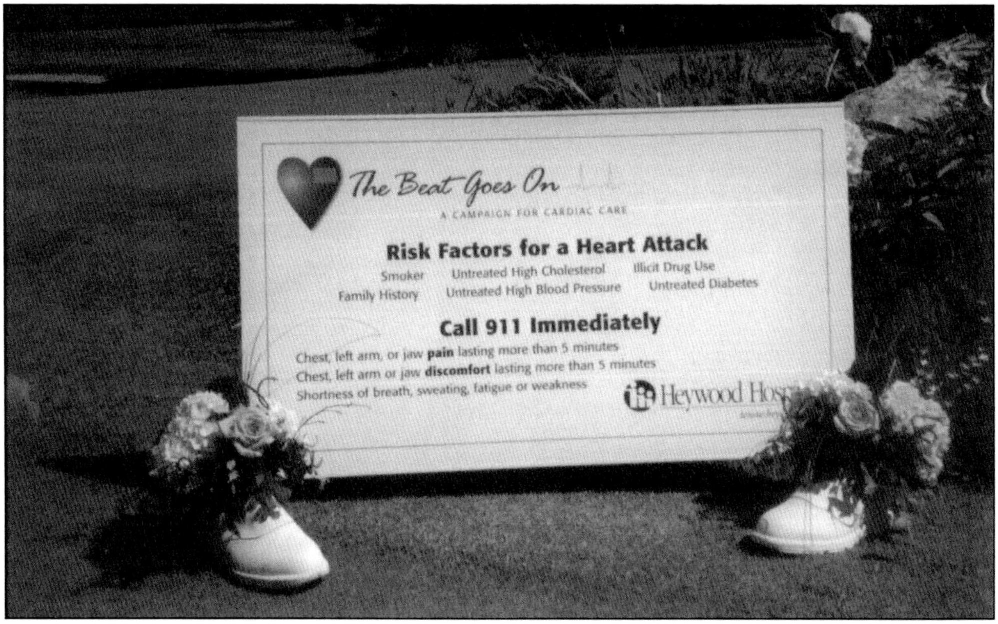
The Beat Goes On
A CAMPAIGN FOR CARDIAC CARE
Risk Factors for a Heart Attack
Smoker
Untreated High Cholesterol
Illicit Drug Use
Family History
Untreated High Blood Pressure
Untreated Diabetes
Call 911 Immediately
Chest, left arm, or jaw pain lasting more than 5 minutes
Chest, left arm or jaw discomfort lasting more than 5 minutes
Shortness of breath, sweating, fatigue or weakness

The years 1999 through 2001 were dedicated to the memory of Tom Kelly. A Spirit of America campaign in 2002 followed the September 11, 2001, terrorist attacks. The Gift of Hope campaign singled out the oncology unit and the Caring Community campaign the mental health unit. This is the decorative display for The Beat Goes On campaign benefiting the Cardiac Rehabilitation Center.

Ten

The Next Century

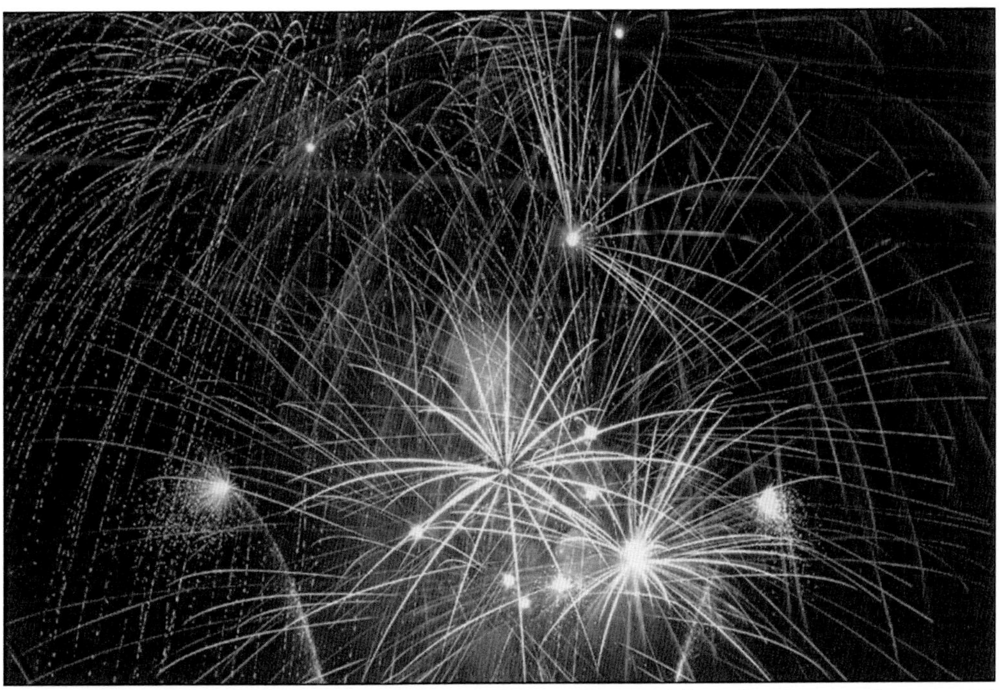

In June 2007, the 100th anniversary of Heywood Hospital was celebrated with a grand centennial ball and other festivities. Historic displays highlighted the story of the hospital. Entertainment included a video highlighting the successes, dancing, and general merriment. In conjunction with Mount Wachusett Community College, the hospital also hosted a community picnic with games, bands, parachutes, and spectacular fireworks to celebrate 100 years of community service.

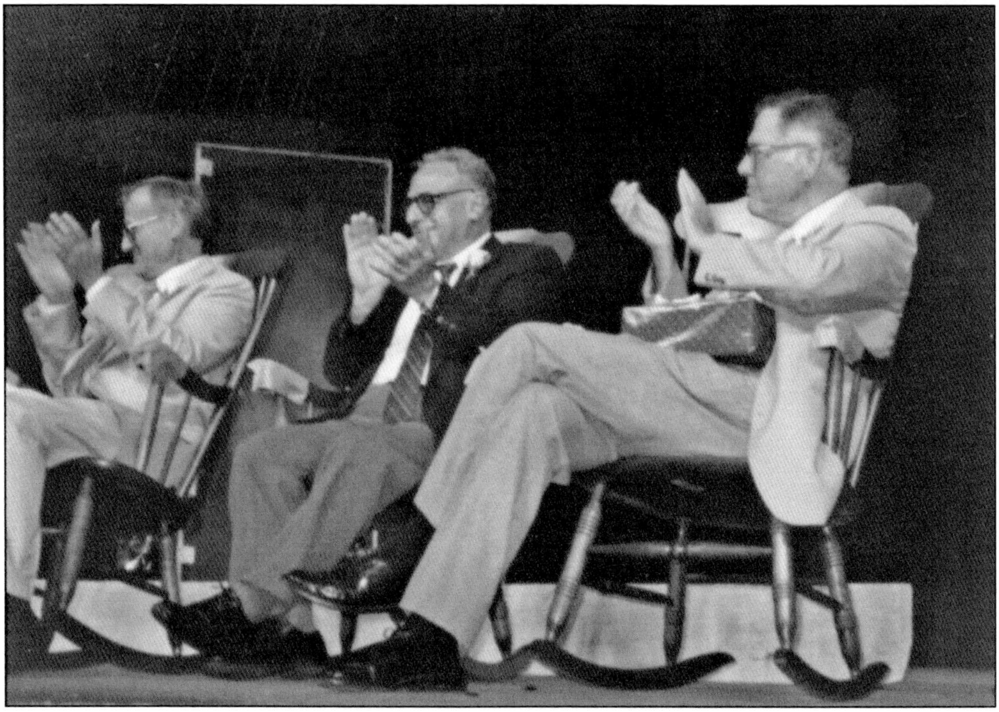

Retirement celebrations for members of the Heywood Hospital family have been a tradition at the hospital. The medical staff and employees never missed an opportunity to celebrate and perform—they loved it. An added benefit was that fellow employees and physicians often interacted in a different venue, encouraging closer ties. Shown in their rocking chairs from left to right, Dr. Max Frei, Dr. Rocco Raduazo, and Dr. Tom Tracy enjoy the festivities hosted by their colleagues at their triple retirement party held at neighboring Mount Wachusett Community College in 1989. The medical staff dressed up as the Village People and performed the song "YMCA." Below are physicians Owen Christensen in scuba gear (second from left), David Havlin as a construction worker (fourth from left), Tim Eddy as a cyclist (second from right), and John Harrington as an American Indian (right). (Both, courtesy of Glenna Mazure, RN.)

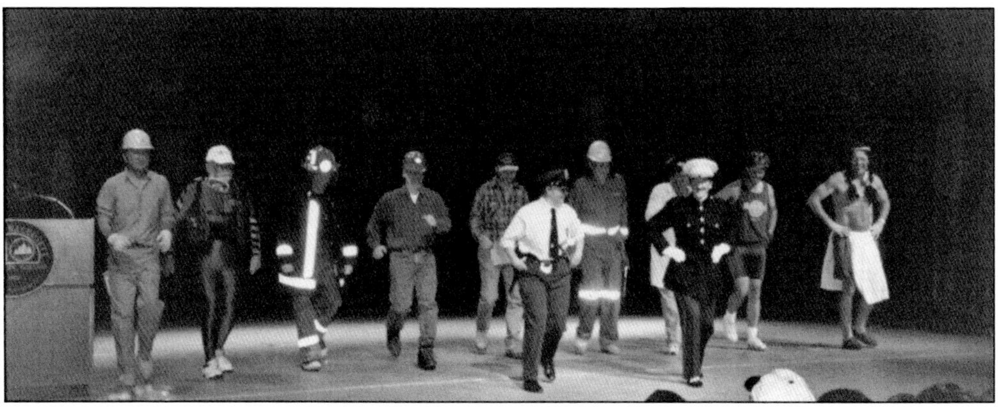

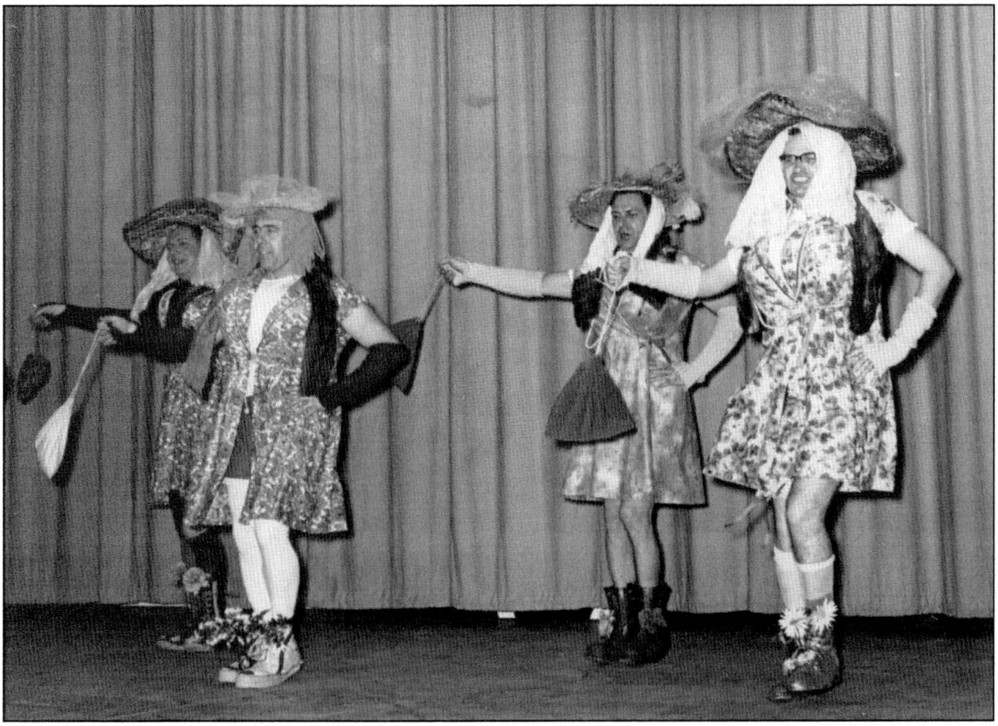

As is evidenced here, as early as the 1960s, Dr. Jim Faust (right) and friends would seize every opportunity to ham it up. Here, they dance at the Hospital Aid Association fundraiser *High Fever Follies*. The flowers added to the laces of the work boots are a nice touch. Seen below several decades later, his colleagues continue the tradition. Posing for the camera at Faust's 2004 retirement party held at Montachusett Regional Vocational Technical School in Fitchburg, Massachusetts, are, from left to right, physicians John Skrzypczak, Tariq Malik, John Harrington, Andrea Damour, Jim Tierney, Kelton Burbank, Tim Eddy, and Lisa Rembetsy-Brown.

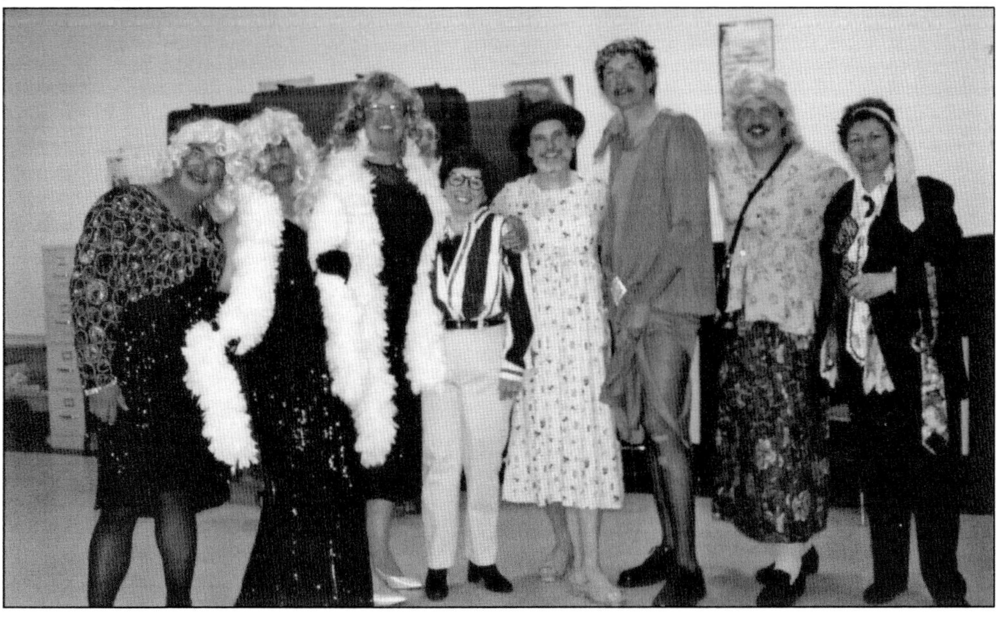

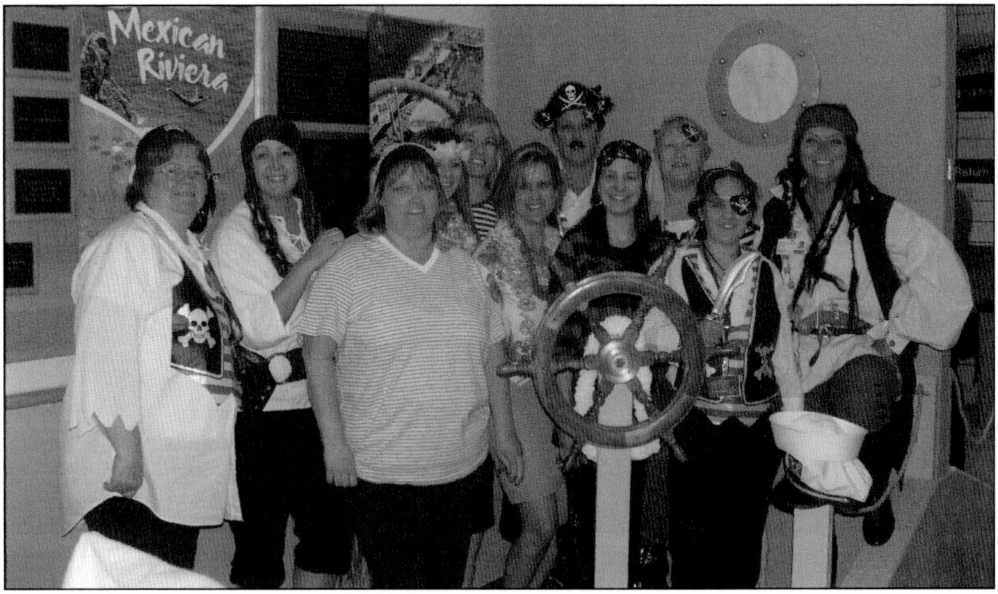

Fundraisers and festivities over the last century highlight Heywood Hospital's strong connection to the Heywood community. Employees and physicians recall annual Hospital Week celebrations with activities like hula dancing lessons and game show reenactments, including *Are You Smarter Than a 5th Grader*. One physician recalls volunteering as a "dunking tank target" for a hospital fundraiser. Other employees reminisce about annual summer outings to the Otter River Sportsmen's Club. Above, a group of Heywood Hospital "pirates" absconds with the ship during a Hospital Week activity. Below, Dr. Donald Miller is playing softball at an annual summer outing. (Below, courtesy of Glenna H. Mazure, RN.)

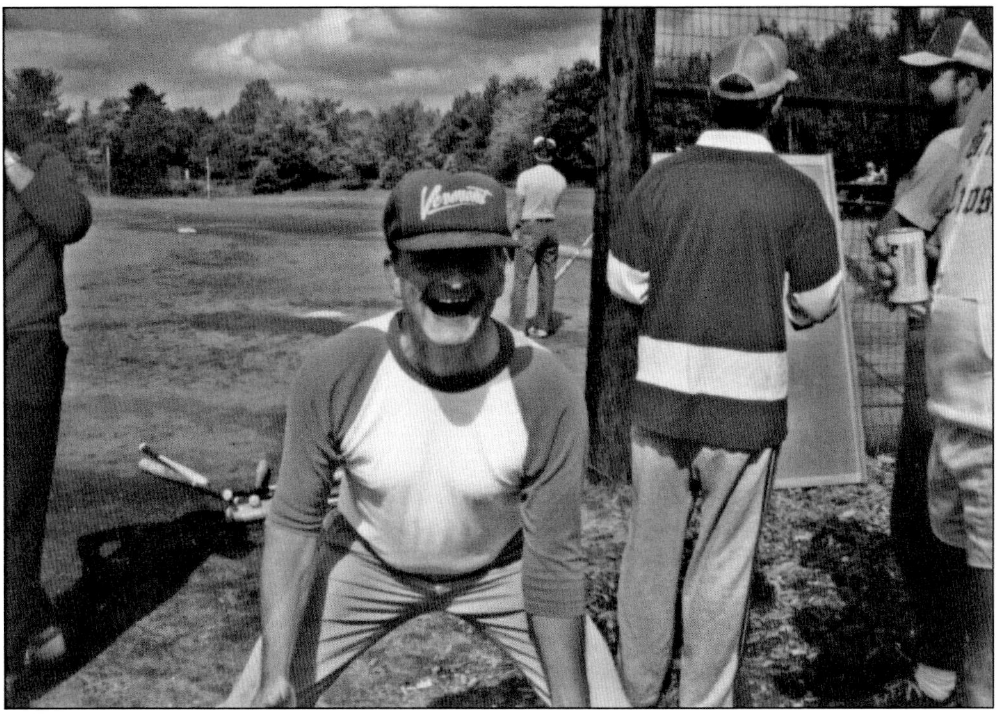

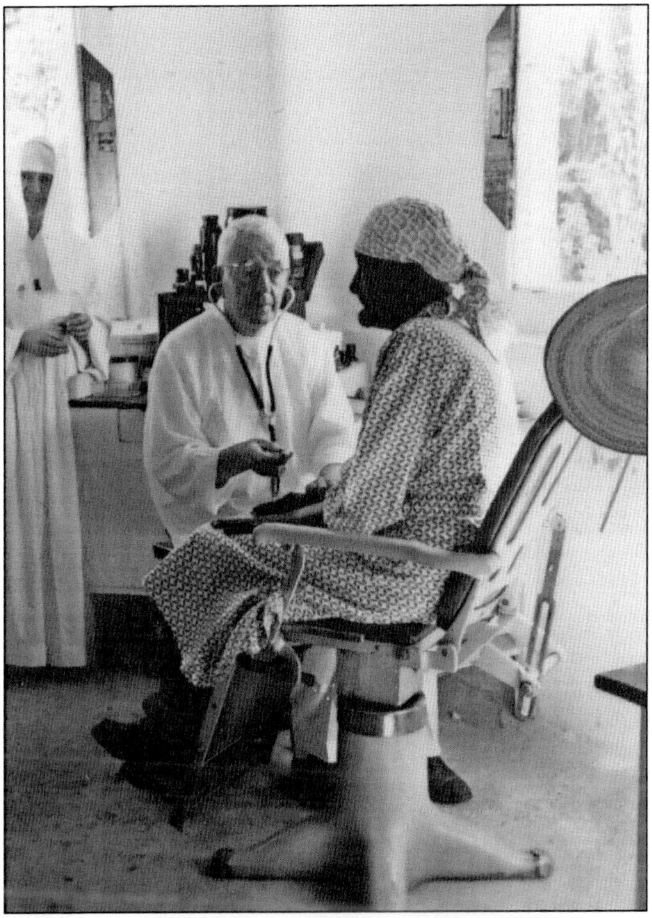

An interesting parallel is that of the humanitarian efforts of a past Heywood Hospital physician and a present one. Dr. Alfred LaChance was a surgeon at the newly established Henry Heywood Memorial Hospital in 1907 and eventually became the chief of surgery. These images were taken between 1948 and 1951 when LaChance embarked on humanitarian medical aid missions in Les Cayes, Haiti. There, LaChance provided much-needed medical care to 40–50 patients per day. Many travelled 50 miles over mountainous terrain to reach the care of the *docteur Americain*. In 2006, Heywood Hospital pediatrician Dr. John Mulqueen and his wife, Paula, founded Forward in Health, a nonprofit organization providing a permanent medical presence in the Les Cayes region of Haiti. (Both, courtesy of Louise G. Plamondon.)

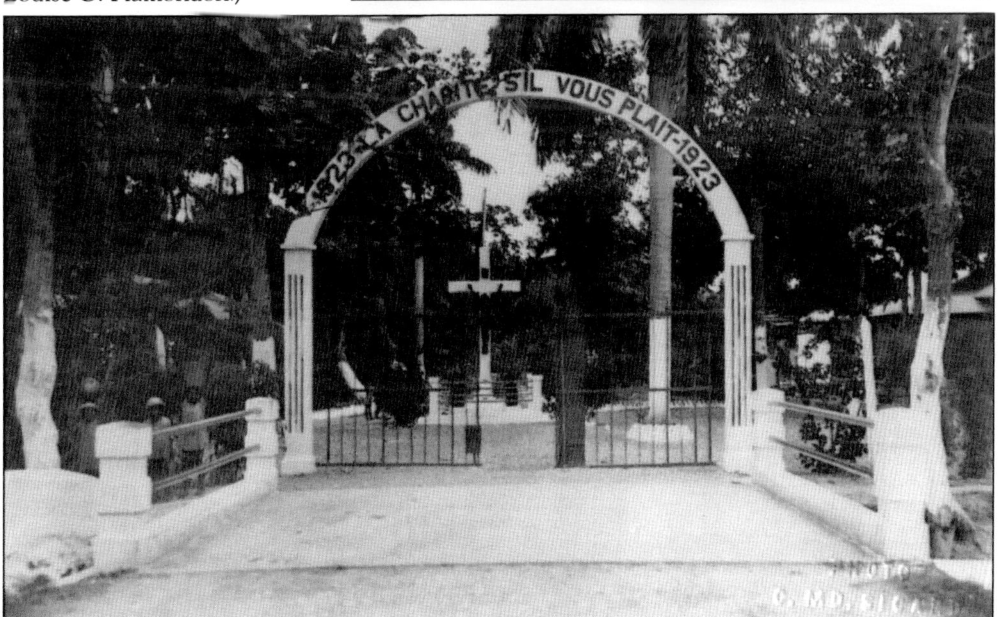

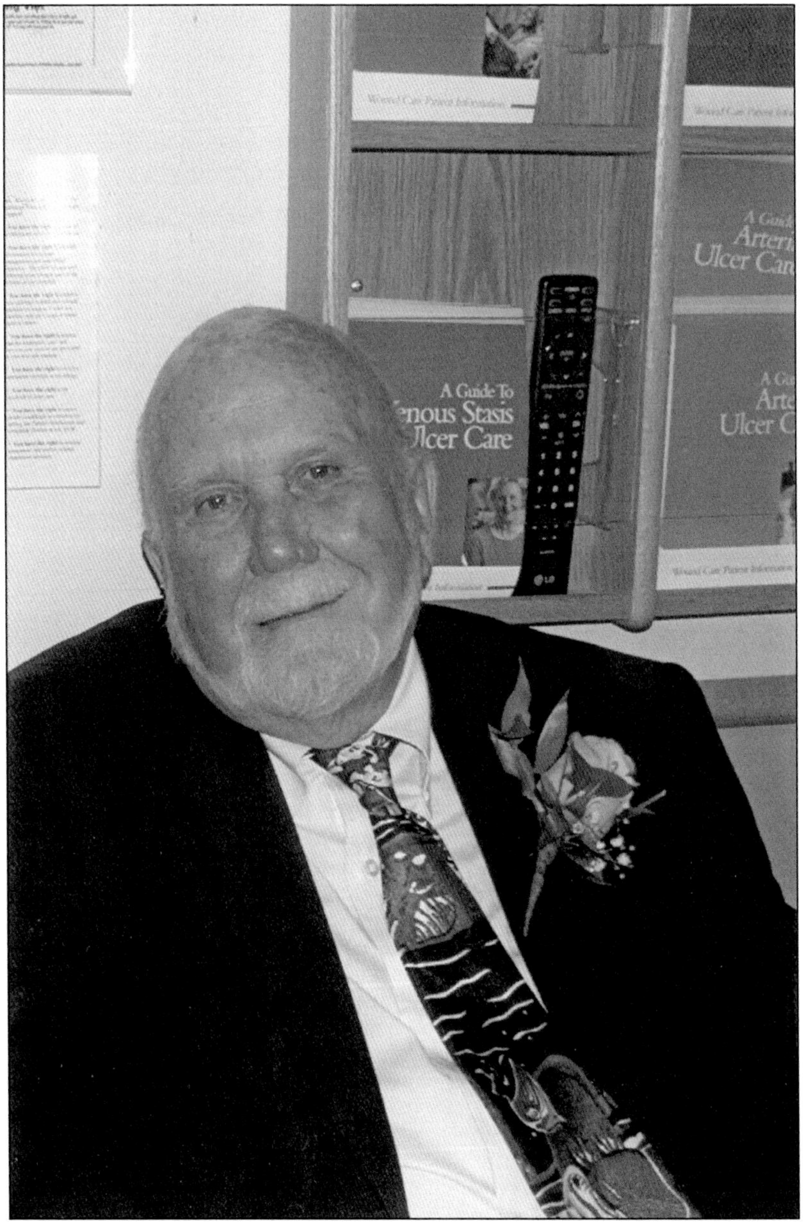

With an eye on the future, Heywood Hospital continues to add and improve services for its patients. Heywood Hospital is the only hospital in the area that offers hyperbaric oxygen therapy, greatly thanks to the vision and persistence of internist Dr. Owen Christensen. For over 50 years, Christensen has been a well-loved member of the Heywood family by his patients and colleagues alike. A recreational scuba diver, Christensen was aware of the benefits of oxygen-rich therapy for treating wounds and other conditions. While in a pressurized chamber, the patient breathes 100 percent oxygen. Oxygen concentration is increased in all body tissues, stimulating healing. The epitome of a lifelong learner, Christensen well deserved the recent dedication ceremony that honored him in the founding of Heywood Hospital's Center for Wound Care and Hyperbaric Medicine. The center adds yet another way in which local residents can be treated in their own community, as opposed to having to travel outside the area.

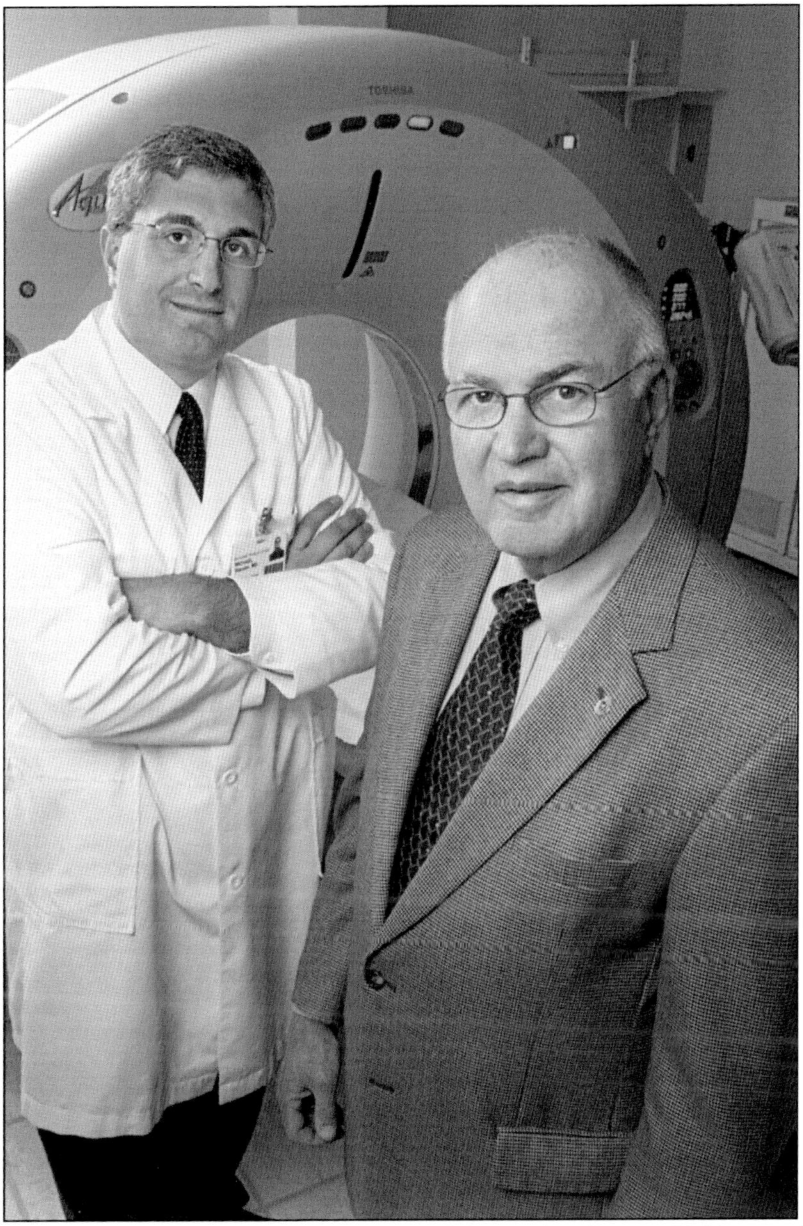

Heywood Hospital trustee and longtime supporter of the Gardner Rotary Club's annual auction, James Garrison (right) successfully bid on a cardiac assessment screening utilizing a newly installed 64-slice CT scanner at Heywood Hospital. This technology allows for noninvasive cardiac testing and identification of arterial blockages. After meeting with cardiologist Dr. Michael Stauder, Garrison underwent a comprehensive cardiac evaluation and scanning with the 64-slice machine and proceeded home. Later that evening, he was surprised to hear the news from Stauder that the scanner had revealed significant blockages in several arteries. Within a couple of days, Garrison underwent the necessary procedures to open the blocked arteries and reported feeling better than he had in a long time. Glad he placed that auction bid and crediting the cardiac care equipment available locally at Heywood Hospital, Garrison stated, "The cardiac CT at Heywood saved my life."

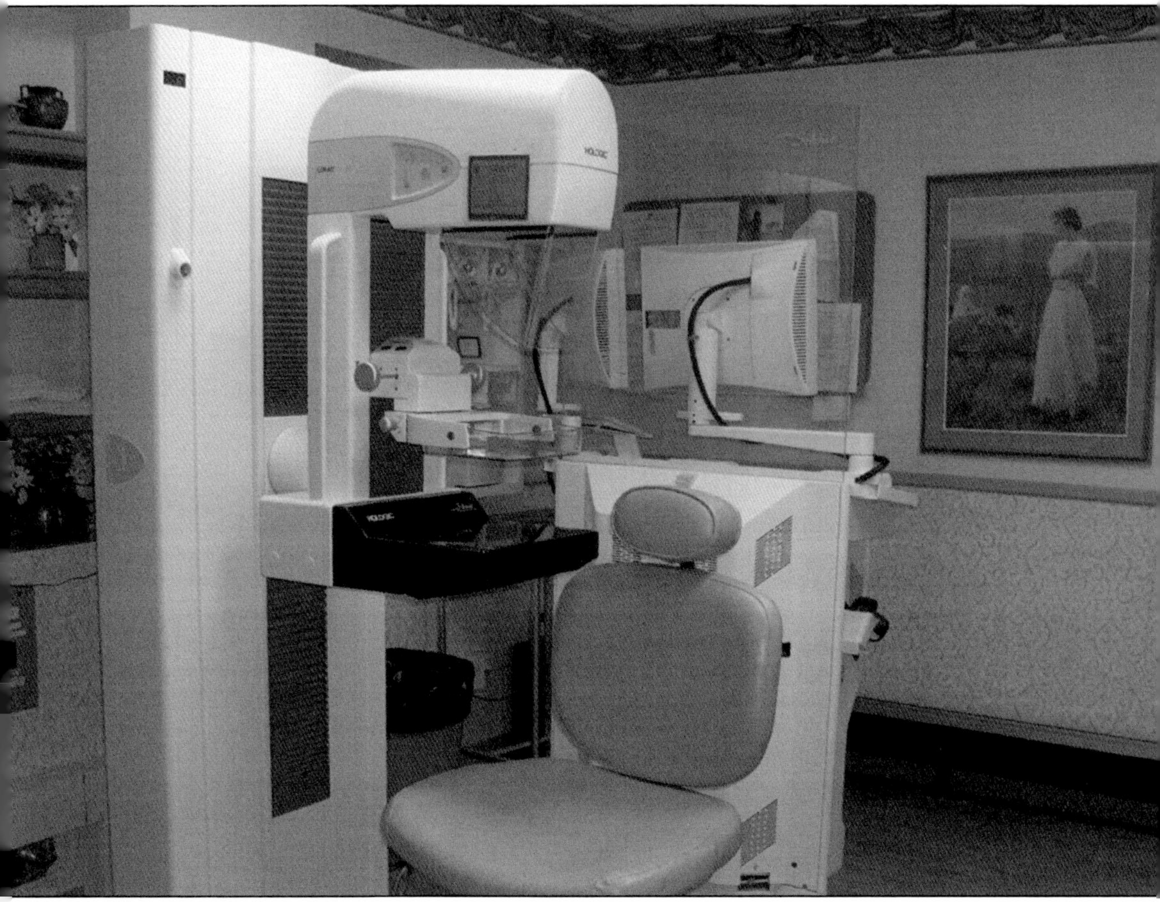

Here is a digital mammography machine. Mammograms were initiated at Heywood Hospital in the early 1970s. To perform mammograms, industrial film requiring a very long exposure was used. Mammography has come a long way to the current use of digital mammography. Heywood Hospital now utilizes digital mammography for the prevention and detection of breast cancers. The mammography chair in this photograph was donated by the Hospital Aid Association. Capsule endoscopy is another cutting-edge technology now offered by Heywood Hospital. This procedure utilizes a camera inside of a capsule that the patient swallows. During the next eight hours, the camera transmits images to a data recorder. Special software allows the physician to carefully review the collected images and identify any abnormalities. Because this noninvasive procedure is now available at Heywood Hospital, patients are able to remain in their community, going about their normal routine while the exam is being conducted.

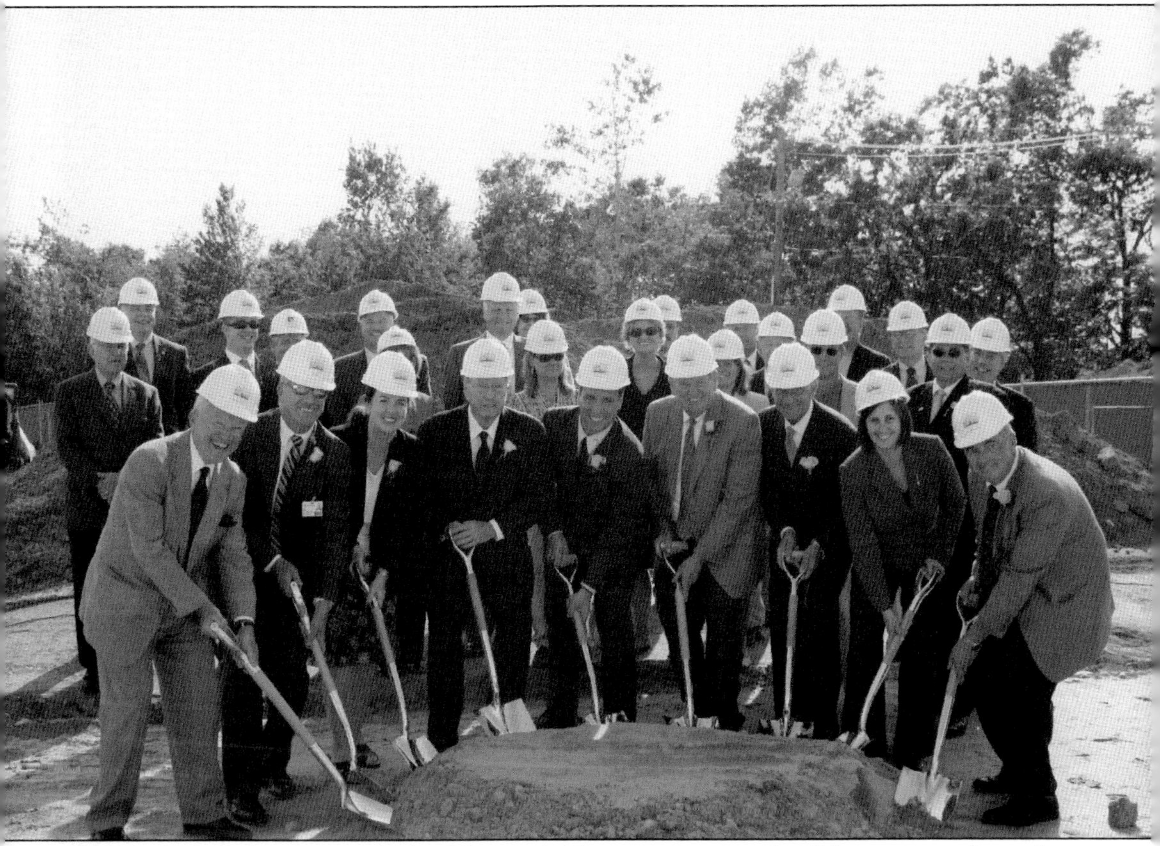

With the knowledge that in the health care field one cannot stand still but must go forward, Heywood Hospital launched a $36 million project for the Watkins Center for Emergency and Acute Care in 2008. This addition provided a wide array of new and improved services for the community. The Next Century campaign raised $10 million over three years. The Heywood Hospital family of trustees, employees, physicians, and Hospital Aid Association contributed $1.5 million. Additional contributions included $350,000 from the Robinson Broadhurst Foundation of Winchendon, Massachusetts, $1.15 million from community members, and $7 million from the E.G. Watkins Family Foundation. This image was taken at the groundbreaking celebration in June 2009. Pictured from left to right in the front row are Rep. Bob Rice, CEO and president Dan Moen, Karen Watkins, Chris Watkins, Mayor Mark Hawke, Dr. Jim Faust, chairman of the board Dan Asquino, Rep. Jennifer Flanagan, and Dr. John Skrzypczak.

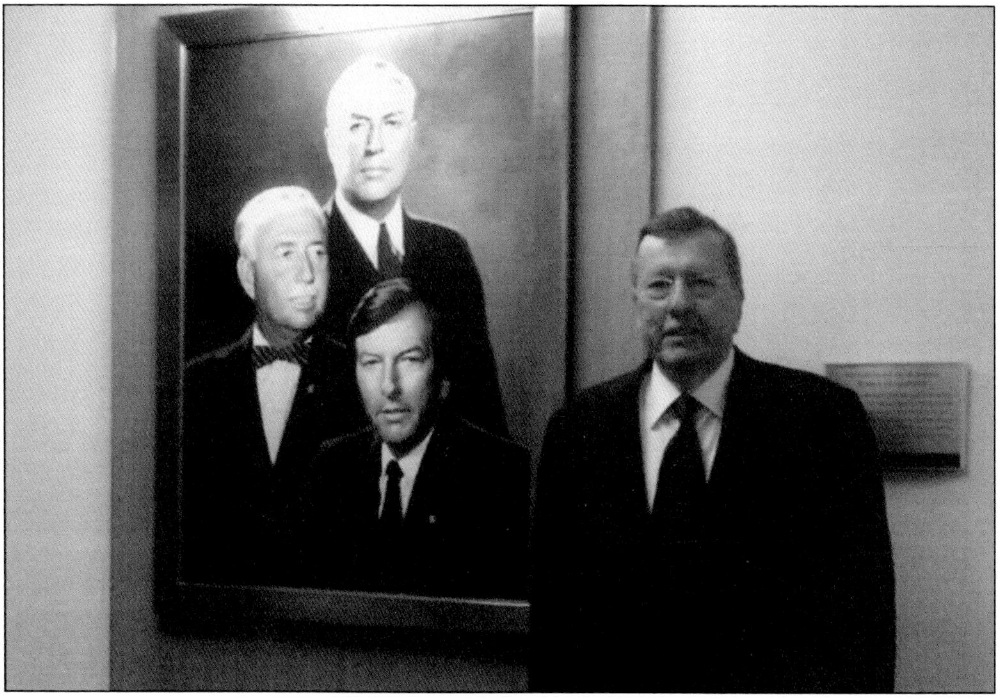

Chris Watkins is shown standing next to a portrait of him and his family. The Watkinses have been exemplary philanthropic friends to Heywood Hospital over three generations, playing major roles in the growth of the hospital. The Watkins Center for Emergency and Acute Care opened in November 2010. The complex is 72,000 square feet, increasing the size of the hospital by one-third. An emergency room and a radiology unit occupy the ground floor. Watkins I houses the intensive care, telemetry, and surgical units. Watkins II has a 25-bed medical surgical unit. Below is the front facade of the new Watkins Center for Emergency and Acute Care.

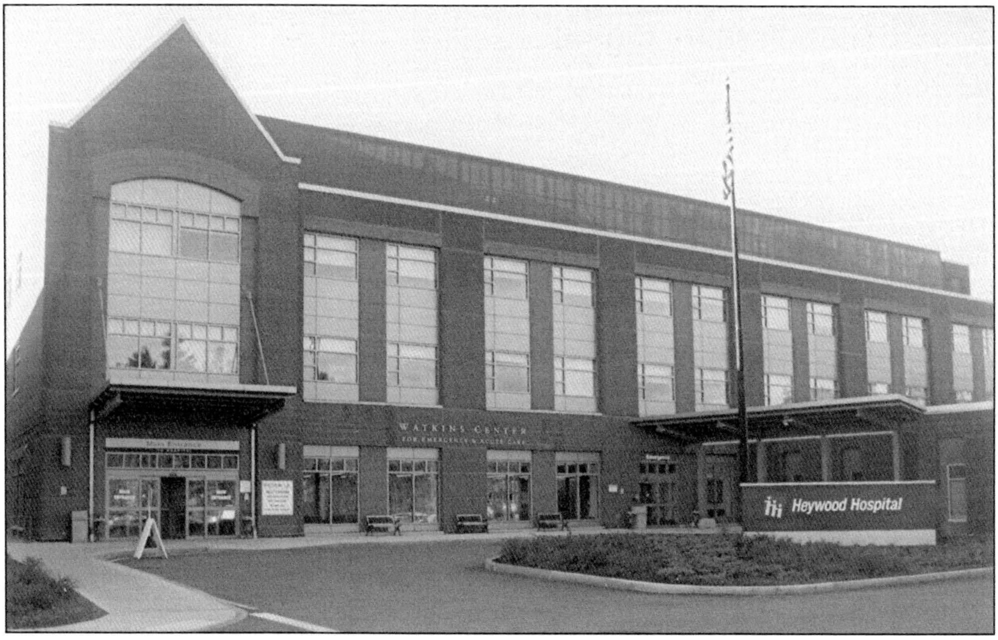

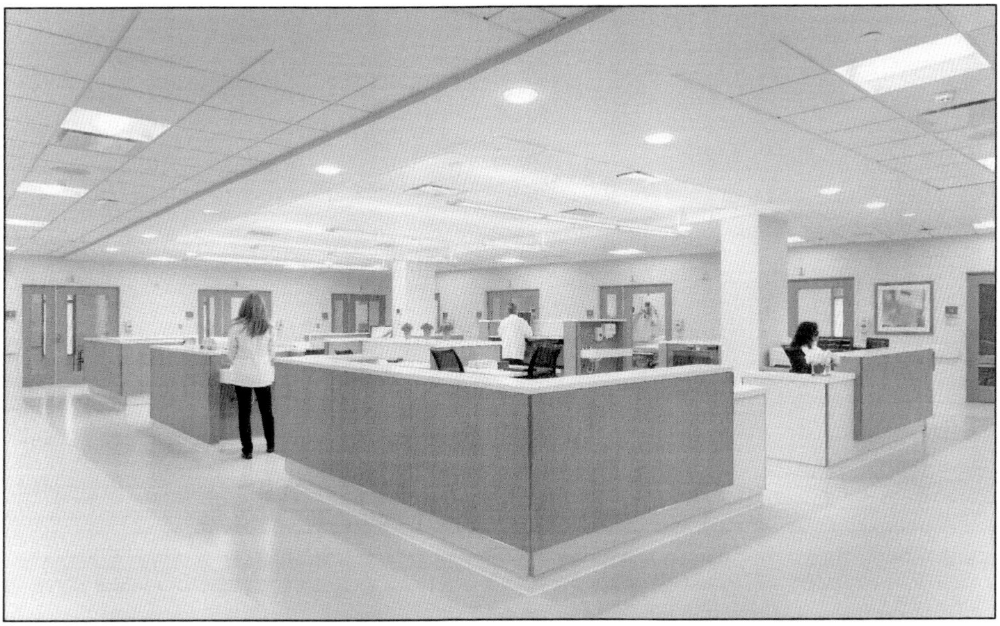

This new Watkins Center for Emergency and Acute Care doubles the number of patient exam rooms of the 1993 emergency department. The former emergency department had 10 exam rooms and a capacity of 10,000–15,000 patient visits per year, not nearly enough for the 21,000 visits the emergency department received. Today's emergency department has 18 exam rooms plus two trauma rooms, accommodating up to 30,000 patient visits annually.

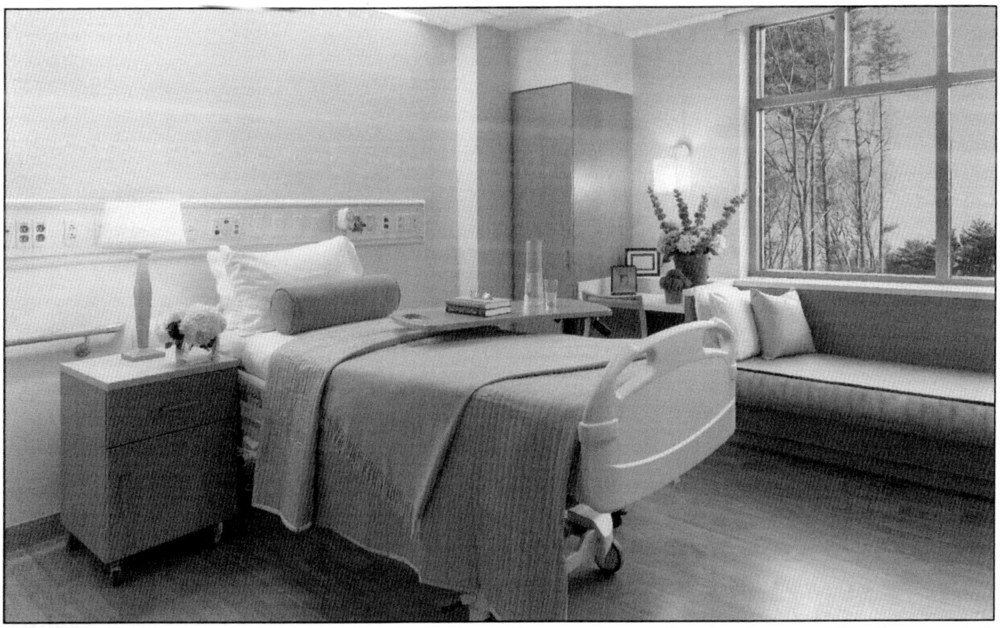

The surgical and medical patient rooms are all private rooms and are patient and family oriented. Pullout daybeds in each room allow family members to stay overnight with their loved ones. Patient servers—cabinets stocked with the most frequently needed supplies—are just steps from the bedside and improve patient care and efficiency. The 32-inch, flat-screen televisions are appreciated, as are the family conference rooms with computer capabilities.

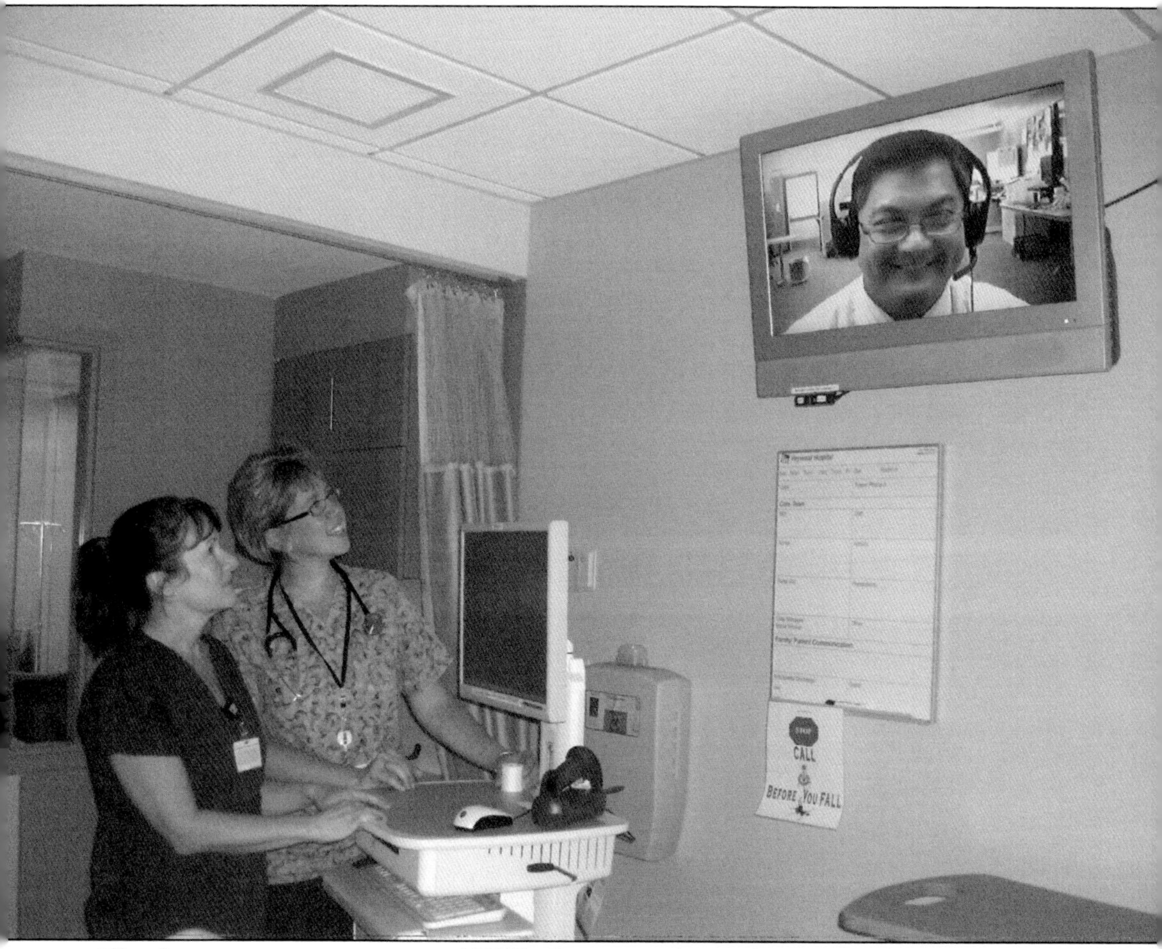

The electronic intensive care unit (eICU) allows critical-care physicians and nurse practitioners at University of Massachusetts Memorial Health Care (UMMHC) to monitor Heywood Hospital patients in the intensive care unit, providing additional expert support. The monitoring system that tracks heart rhythm, pulse, blood pressure, and oxygen level at Heywood Hospital in Gardner is continuously monitored at UMMHC in Worcester. The eICU provides support and expertise for the Heywood Hospital physicians and nurses. If questions or problems arise, the UMMHC critical-care physician is immediately available. Using a television screen, two-way communication and visualization is achieved. The critical-care physician can observe the patient and even measure the diameter of the patient's pupils. Thus, the eICU literally provides another pair of eyes to closely watch Heywood Hospital's ICU patients. The eICU allows more patients to be cared for at their local hospital. Here, nurses consult with the critical-care physician at UMMHC visible on the television screen.

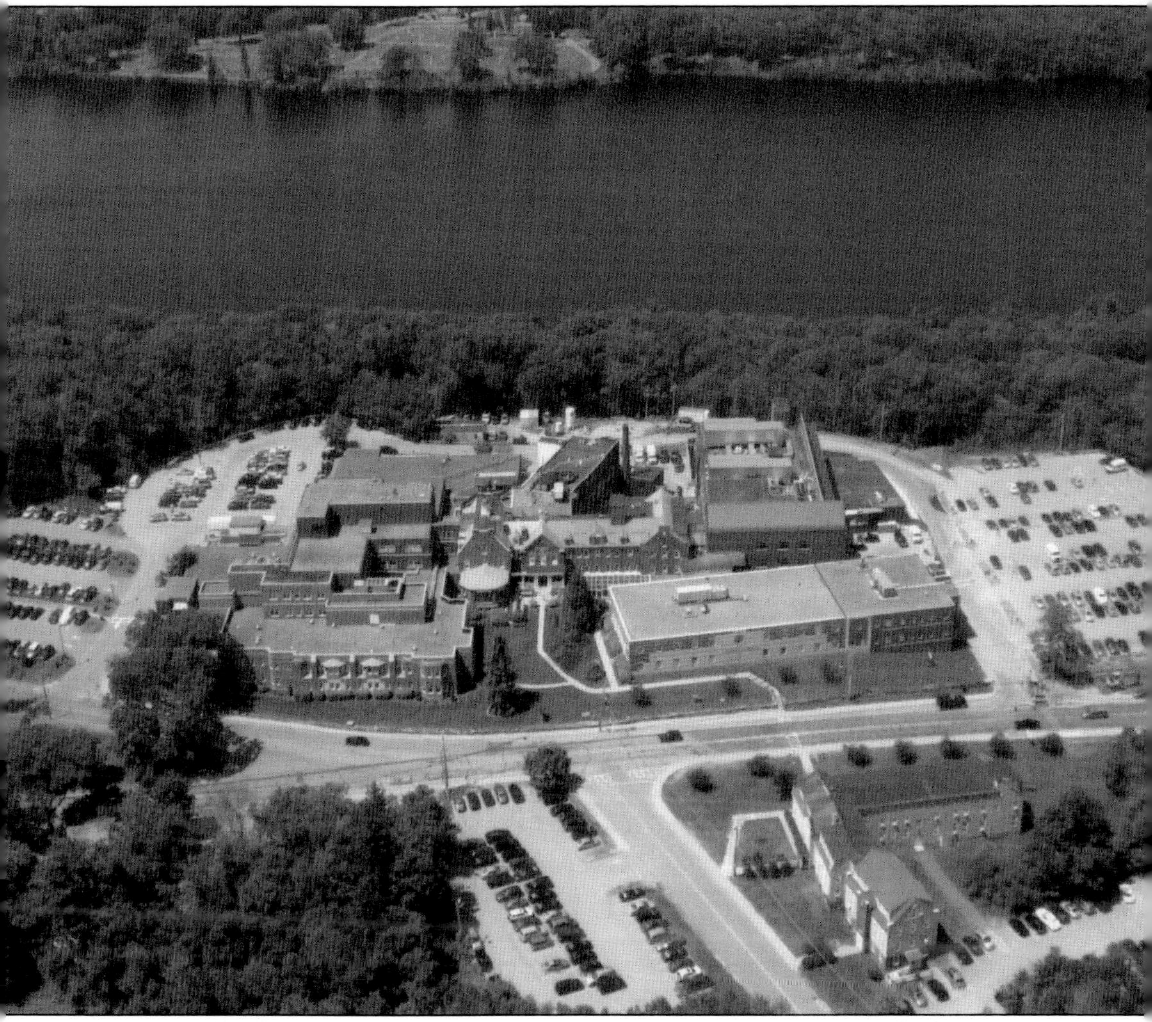

Henry Heywood wished to spare his factory workers from travelling to Boston for medical care. The result was the establishment of Henry Heywood Memorial Hospital in 1907. Today, area residents can still remain local for their medical care thanks to the eICU and other specialized services available at Heywood Hospital. This aerial view looks west toward Crystal Lake, showing the hospital in its entirety. Recessed in the center is the original 1907 hospital with its white-pillared porch and its early additions. The old Heywood farmhouse, first converted to the nursing school and then used as the administration building, is visible at lower right. Crossing Green Street in the left foreground is the maternity center, Ambulatory Care Center, and oncology unit. To its rear are the Favor Wing, the radiology unit, and the cafeteria. The Medical Arts Building is in the right foreground. Finally, to its rear are the 2010 main entrance and Watkins Emergency and Acute Care Center. The realization of Henry Heywood's wish for a local hospital continues to persevere a century later. (Courtesy of Dr. John Skrzypczak.)